Delivery After Previous Cesarean

Guest Editors

CAROLINE SIGNORE, MD, MPH
MARK B. LANDON, MD

CLINICS IN PERINATOLOGY

www.perinatology.theclinics.com

Consulting Editor

LUCKY JAIN, MD, MBA

June 2011 • Volume 38 • Number 2

SAUNDERS an imprint of ELSEVIER, Inc.

W.B. SAUNDERS COMPANY
A Division of Elsevier Inc.

Elsevier, Inc. • 1600 John F. Kennedy Blvd. • Suite 1800 • Philadelphia, PA 19103-2899

http://www.theclinics.com

CLINICS IN PERINATOLOGY Volume 38, Number 2
June 2011 ISSN 0095-5108, ISBN-13: 978-1-4557-0485-9

Editor: Kerry Holland
Developmental Editor: Teia Stone

Clinics in Perinatology (ISSN 0095-5108) is published quarterly by Elsevier Inc., 360 Park Avenue South, New York, NY 10010-1710. Months of issue are March, June, September, and December. Business and Editorial Offices: 1600 John F. Kennedy Blvd., Ste. 1800, Philadelphia, PA 19103-2899. Customer Service Office: 3251 Riverport Lane, Maryland Heights, MO 63043. Periodicals postage paid at New York, NY and additional mailing offices. Subscription prices are $256.00 per year (US individuals), $382.00 per year (US institutions), $306.00 per year (Canadian individuals), $485.00 per year (Canadian institutions), $376.00 per year (foreign individuals), $485.00 per year (foreign institutions) $122.00 per year (US students), and $176.00 per year (Canadian and foreign students). Foreign air speed delivery is included in all Clinics subscription prices. All prices are subject to change without notice. **POSTMASTER:** Send address changes to *Clinics in Perinatology*, Elsevier Health Sciences Division, Subscription Customer Service, 3251 Riverport Lane, Maryland Heights, MO 63043. **Customer Service: Telephone: 1-800-654-2452** (U.S. and Canada); **1-314-447-8871** (outside U.S. and Canada). **Fax: 1-314-447-8029. E-mail: journalscustomerservice-usa@elsevier.com** (for print support); **journalsonlinesupport-usa@elsevier.com** (for online support).

Reprints. For copies of 100 or more, of articles in this publication, please contact the Commercial Reprints Department, Elsevier Inc., 360 Park Avenue South, New York, NY 10010-1710. Tel. (212) 633-3812; Fax: (212) 482-1935; email: reprints@elsevier.com.

Clinics in Perinatology is also published in Spanish by McGraw-Hill Interamericana Editores S.A., P.O. Box 5-237, 06500 Mexico D.F., Mexico.

Clinics in Perinatology is covered in *MEDLINE/PubMed (Index Medicus) Current Contents, Excepta Medica, BIOSIS and ISI/BIOMED.*

Printed and bound by CPI Group (UK) Ltd, Croydon, CR0 4YY
Transferred to Digital Print 2011

Contributors

CONSULTING EDITOR

LUCKY JAIN, MD, MBA
Richard Blumberg Professor and Executive Vice Chairman, Department of Pediatrics, Emory University School of Medicine, Atlanta, Georgia

GUEST EDITORS

CAROLINE SIGNORE, MD, MPH
Program Officer/Project Scientist, Pregnancy and Perinatology Branch, Eunice Kennedy Shriver National Institute of Child Health and Human Development, Bethesda, Maryland

MARK B. LANDON, MD
Richard L. Meiling Professor and Chairman, Department of Obstetrics and Gynecology, Ohio State University College of Medicine, Columbus, Ohio

AUTHORS

MERLYN P. BARRETO, MD
Research Fellow, Discipline of Obstetrics and Gynaecology, Women's and Children's Hospital, The University of Adelaide, North Adelaide, South Australia, Australia

RICHARD BERKOWITZ, MD
Professor of Obstetrics and Gynecology, Director of Quality Improvement, Department of Obstetrics and Gynecology, Columbia University, New York, New York

CLARISSA BONANNO, MD
Assistant Clinical Professor of Obstetrics and Gynecology, Department of Obstetrics and Gynecology, Columbia University, New York, New York

ALISON G. CAHILL, MD
Assistant Professor, Division of Maternal-Fetal Medicine, Department of Obstetrics and Gynecology, Washington University in St Louis, Missouri

AARON B. CAUGHEY, MD, PhD
Professor and Chair, Department of Obstetrics and Gynecology, Oregon Health & Science University, Portland, Oregon

YVONNE W. CHENG, MD, MPH
Assistant Professor, Division of Maternal-Fetal Medicine, Department of Obstetrics, Gynecology and Reproductive Sciences, University of California San Francisco, San Francisco, California

FRANK A. CHERVENAK, MD
Given Foundation Professor and Chairman, Department of Obstetrics and
Gynecology, New York-Presbyterian Hospital – Weill Cornell Medical College,
New York, New York

MARILEE CLAUSING, RN, BSN, JD
Partner and Trial Attorney in the Chicago Law Firm of Anderson, Anderson,
Rasor & Partners, LLP, Chicago, Illinois

EUGENE DECLERCQ, PhD
Assistant Dean for Doctoral Education and Professor, Department of Community Health
Sciences, Boston University School of Public Health, Boston, Massachusetts

JODIE M. DODD, PhD, FRANZCOG, CMFM
Professor, Discipline of Obstetrics and Gynaecology, Women's and Children's Hospital,
The University of Adelaide, North Adelaide, South Australia, Australia

MITZI DONABEL A. GO, MD
Fellow of Neonatal and Perinatal Medicine, Division of Neonatology, Department of
Pediatrics, Oregon Health & Science University, Portland, Oregon

KAREN B. EDEN, PhD
Associate Professor, Department of Medical Informatics and Clinical Epidemiology,
Oregon Evidence-based Practice Center, Oregon Health and Science University,
Portland, Oregon

CATHY EMEIS, PhD
Assistant Professor, Nurse-Midwifery Program, School of Nursing, Oregon
Health & Science University, Portland, Oregon

MOSHE FRIDMAN, PhD
AMF Consulting, Inc, Los Angeles, California

KIMBERLY D. GREGORY, MD, MPH
Department of Obstetrics & Gynecology, Burns Allen Research Institute, Cedars-Sinai
Medical Center; Department of Obstetrics & Gynecology, David Geffen School of
Medicine; Department of Community Health Sciences, UCLA School of Public Health,
Los Angeles, California

ROSALIE M. GRIVELL, BSc, BMBS, FRANZCOG
Senior Lecturer, Discipline of Obstetrics and Gynaecology, Women's and Children's
Hospital, The University of Adelaide, North Adelaide, South Australia, Australia

JEANNE-MARIE GUISE, MD, MPH
Associate Professor, Division of Maternal-Fetal Medicine, Departments of Obstetrics
and Gynecology, Medical Informatics and Clinical Epidemiology, and Public Health and
Preventive Medicine, Oregon Evidence-based Practice Center, Oregon Health and
Science University; Quality & Safety for Women's Services, Health Services and
Outcomes Research, Oregon BIRCWH K12, Comparative Effectiveness K12 & KM1,
Institute for Patient Centered Comparative Effectiveness, State Obstetric and Pediatric
Research Collaborative (STORC), OHSU Center of Excellence in Women's Health,
Oregon Health & Science University Hospital, Portland, Oregon

ANDREW D. HULL, MD
Professor of Clinical Reproductive Medicine, Division of Perinatal Medicine, Department of Reproductive Medicine, University of California San Diego, La Jolla, San Diego, California

TEKOA L. KING, CNM, MPH
Clinical Professor, Department of Obstetrics, Gynecology and Reproductive Medicine; Deputy Editor, Journal of Midwifery & Women's Health, University of California San Francisco, California

LISA M. KORST, MD, PhD
Department of Obstetrics & Gynecology, Keck School of Medicine, University of Southern California, Los Angeles; Senior Scientist, Childbirth Research Associates, LLC, North Hollywood, California

MARIAN MACDORMAN, PhD
Senior Statistician, Division of Vital Statistics, Reproductive Statistics Branch, National Center for Health Statistics, Centers for Disease Control and Prevention, Hyattsville, Maryland

NICOLE MARSHALL, MD
Maternal-Fetal Medicine Fellow, Division of Maternal-Fetal Medicine, Department of Obstetrics and Gynecology, Oregon Health & Science University, Portland, Oregon

LAURENCE B. MCCULLOUGH, PhD
Dalton Tomlin Chair in Medical Ethics and Health Policy, Center for Medical Ethics and Health Policy, Baylor College of Medicine, Houston, Texas

FAY MENACKER, DrPH, CPNP
Senior Nurse, Maternal and Child Health, Social & Scientific Systems, Inc, Silver Spring, Maryland

THOMAS R. MOORE, MD
Professor and Chair, Department of Reproductive Medicine, University of California San Diego, La Jolla, San Diego, California

JOSEF NEU, MD
Professor of Pediatrics, Division of Neonatology, Department of Pediatrics; Director, Neonatology Fellowship Training Program, University of Florida, Gainesville, Florida

LEONARDO PEREIRA, MD
Assistant Professor, Division of Maternal-Fetal Medicine, Department of Obstetrics and Gynecology, Oregon Health & Science University, Portland, Oregon

JEFFREY P. PHELAN, MD, JD
Department of Obstetrics and Gynecology, Citrus Valley Medical Center, City of Industry, West Covina, California

JONA RUSHING, MD
Fellow, Division of Maternal Fetal Medicine, Department of Obstetrics and Gynecology, University of Florida, Gainesville, Florida

ROBERT L. SCHELONKA, MD
Associate Professor, Department of Pediatrics; Chief, Division of Neonatology, Oregon Health & Science University, Portland, Oregon

ANTHONY L. SHANKS, MD
Assistant Professor, Division of Maternal-Fetal Medicine, Department of Obstetrics
and Gynecology, Washington University in St Louis, St Louis, Missouri

CAROLYN M. ZELOP, MD
Visiting Associate Professor of Obstetrics and Gynecology, Harvard University School of
Medicine, Division Director of Maternal Fetal Medicine, Beth Israel Deaconess Medical
Center, Boston, Massachusetts

Contents

Cesarean delivery is the most common major surgical procedure for women in the United States, with 1.4 million surgeries annually. In 2008, nearly one-third (32.3%) of US births were by cesarean delivery. Cesarean delivery rates have increased rapidly in the United States in recent years because of an increasing primary cesarean delivery rate and a declining vaginal birth after cesarean (VBAC) rate. In 2007, the VBAC rate was 8.3% in a 22-state reporting area. The US VBAC rate was lowest among 14 industrialized countries; 3 countries had VBAC rates greater than 50%.

The use of trial of labor after cesarean (TOLAC) has declined in the last decade, and the clinical risks of TOLAC remain low. Nonclinical factors continue to affect women's access to TOLAC. This article considers 5 categories of factors that seem to be influencing rates of TOLAC and vaginal birth after cesarean: opinion leaders and professional guidelines, hospital facilities and cesarean availability, reimbursement for providing TOLAC, medical liability, and patient-level factors. An evidence base and strategies to provide guidance to create a safe environment for vaginal birth after cesarean are needed. Obstetric information systems are critical to this effort.

History has always been a series of pendulum swings, and there is perhaps no better example in obstetrics than that of vaginal birth after cesarean. Vaginal birth after cesarean (VBAC) rates rose steadily in the early 1990s. However, VBAC rates have declined dramatically over recent years, while the cesarean delivery rate has continued to rise unabated. Many physicians and hospitals are no longer offering trial of labor after cesarean, largely because of medicolegal concerns. This article explores the medical and legal risks of trial of labor after cesarean.

In 2010, a National Institutes of Health Consensus Panel and the American College of Obstetricians and Gynecologists issued updated statements on trial of labor after cesarean delivery (TOLAC). This article presents an ethical framework for the informed consent process for TOLAC. Three conclusions are reached. For women with one previous low transverse incision, TOLAC and elective repeat cesarean delivery should be offered. Obstetricians should recommend against TOLAC when a pregnant woman has had a previous classical incision. TOLAC after two previous low transverse incisions may be offered provided that the informed consent process presents the uncertainties of the evidence.

Cesarean delivery rates in the United States have reached an all-time high. The current rate of 31% is 6 times higher than the 1970s rate. Many factors including physician preference and hospital accessibility account for this trend. A decreased vaginal birth after cesarean (VBAC) rate and an increased repeat cesarean rate have important consequences for women in future pregnancies. Because of these considerations, VBAC has been an important issue within the obstetric community for over 3 decades. Identifying the best candidates for VBAC using factors available to the obstetrician can increase the VBAC success rate while minimizing maternal morbidity.

Women who undergo a trial of labor after a previous cesarean delivery (TOLAC) have special needs prenatally and during the intrapartum period. Counseling about the choice of TOLAC versus an elective repeat cesarean delivery involves complex statistical concepts. Prenatal counseling that is patient centered, individualized, and presented in a way that addresses the health literacy and health numeracy of the recipient encompasses best practices that support patient decision making. Evidence-based practices during labor that support vaginal birth and increase patient satisfaction are of special value for this population.

Cesarean delivery is common and increasing over time. A prior cesarean birth increases the risk of both elective and emergency cesarean births and uterine rupture in a subsequent pregnancy. A range of factors, including labor characteristics, may influence the risk of these outcomes in the next pregnancy. Intrapartum factors associated with successful vaginal birth and lower risk of uterine rupture include the spontaneous onset of labor and advanced cervical dilatation. In contrast, need for induction and augmentation of labor are both factors associated with an increased likelihood of unsuccessful vaginal birth and risk of uterine rupture.

Uterine rupture, which involves complete separation of the uterine wall, occurs in about 1% of those attempting vaginal birth after cesarean. Because uterine rupture is one of the most significant complications of a trial of labor (TOL) after previous cesarean, identifying those at increased risk of uterine rupture is paramount to the safety of a TOL after previous cesarean birth. It seems that both antepartum demographic characteristics and intrapartum factors modify the risk of uterine rupture. The ability to reliably predict an individual's a priori risk for intrapartum uterine rupture remains a major area of investigation.

Placenta accreta is a significant source of obstetric morbidity and mortality. Its incidence is increasing as a direct consequence of the increasing cesarean section rate, which reflects increased rates of maternal obesity, increased numbers of multiple gestations secondary to assisted reproductive technology, physician concern about litigation for adverse obstetric outcome, and a decline in the use of operative vaginal delivery for both cephalic and breech presentations. Optimum management for most cases requires elective cesarean hysterectomy, ideally performed at about 34 weeks' gestation. A multidisciplinary approach produces the best outcomes.

Nearly 1 in 3 pregnant women in the United States undergo cesarean. This trend is contrary to the national goal of decreasing cesarean delivery in low-risk women. The decline in vaginal birth after cesarean (VBAC) contributes to the continual increase in cesarean deliveries. Prior cesarean delivery is the most common indication for cesarean and accounts for more than one-third of all cesareans. The appropriate use and safety of cesarean and VBAC are of concern not only at the individual patient and clinician level but they also have far-reaching public health and policy implications at the national level.

This article examines data from a recent systematic evidence review on term deliveries conducted for the National Institutes of Health Consensus

GOAL STATEMENT

The goal of *Clinics in Perinatology* is to keep practicing neonatologists and maternal-fetal medicine specialists up to date with current clinical practice in perinatology by providing timely articles reviewing the state of the art in patient care.

ACCREDITATION

The *Clinics in Perinatology* is planned and implemented in accordance with the Essential Areas and Policies of the Accreditation Council for Continuing Medical Education (ACCME) through the joint sponsorship of the University of Virginia School of Medicine and Elsevier. The University of Virginia School of Medicine is accredited by the ACCME to provide continuing medical education for physicians.

The University of Virginia School of Medicine designates this educational activity for a maximum of 15 *AMA PRA Category 1 Credits™* for each issue, 60 credits per year. Physicians should only claim credit commensurate with the extent of their participation in the activity.

The American Medical Association has determined that physicians not licensed in the US who participate in this CME activity are eligible for a maximum of 15 *AMA PRA Category 1 Credits™* for each issue, 60 credits per year.

Credit can be earned by reading the text material, taking the CME examination online at http://www.theclinics.com/home/cme, and completing the evaluation. After taking the test, you will be required to review any and all incorrect answers. Following completion of the test and evaluation, your credit will be awarded and you may print your certificate.

FACULTY DISCLOSURE/CONFLICT OF INTEREST

The University of Virginia School of Medicine, as an ACCME accredited provider, endorses and strives to comply with the Accreditation Council for Continuing Medical Education (ACCME) Standards of Commercial Support, Commonwealth of Virginia statutes, University of Virginia policies and procedures, and associated federal and private regulations and guidelines on the need for disclosure and monitoring of proprietary and financial interests that may affect the scientific integrity and balance of content delivered in continuing medical education activities under our auspices.

The University of Virginia School of Medicine requires that all CME activities accredited through this institution be developed independently and be scientifically rigorous, balanced and objective in the presentation/discussion of its content, theories and practices.

All authors/editors participating in an accredited CME activity are expected to disclose to the readers relevant financial relationships with commercial entities occurring within the past 12 months (such as grants or research support, employee, consultant, stock holder, member of speakers bureau, etc.). The University of Virginia School of Medicine will employ appropriate mechanisms to resolve potential conflicts of interest to maintain the standards of fair and balanced education to the reader. Questions about specific strategies can be directed to the Office of Continuing Medical Education, University of Virginia School of Medicine, Charlottesville, Virginia.

The faculty and staff of the University of Virginia Office of Continuing Medical Education have no financial affiliations to disclose.

The authors/editors listed below have identified no professional or financial affiliations for themselves or their spouse/partner:

Merlyn P. Barreto, MD; Richard Berkowitz, MD; Clarissa Bonanno, MD; Robert Boyle, MD (Test Author); Alison G. Cahill, MD; Yvonne W. Cheng, MD, MPH; Frank A. Chervenak, MD; Marilee Clausing, RN, BSN, JD; Eugene Declercq, PhD; Jodie M. Dodd, PhD, FRANZCOG, CMFM; Karen B. Eden, PhD; Moshe Fridman, PhD; Mitzi Donabel A. Go, MD; Rosalie M. Grivell, BSc, BMBS, FRANZCOG; Jeanne-Marie Guise, MD, MPH; Kerry Holland (Acquisitions Editor); Andrew D. Hull, MD; Lucky Jain, MD, MBA (Consulting Editor); Teoka L. King, CNM, MPH; Lisa M. Korst, MD, PhD; Mark B. Landon, MD (Guest Editor); Marian MacDorman, PhD; Nicole Marshall, MD; Laurence B. McCullough, PhD; Fay Menacker, DrPH, CPNP; Thomas R. Moore, MD; Leonardo Pereira, MD, Jeffrey P. Phelan, MD, JD; Jona Rushing, MD; Robert L. Schelonka, MD; Anthony L. Shanks, MD; and Carolyn M. Zelop, MD.

The authors/editors listed below identified the following professional or financial affiliations for themselves or their spouse/partner:

Aaron B. Caughey, MD, PhD is on the Advisory Committee/Board for Tandem Technology.

Cathy Emeis, PhD is a consultant for InJoy Videos.

Kimberly D. Gregory, MD, MPH is employed by Cedars-Sinai Medical Center.

Josef Neu, MD has a research grant, is on the Advisory Board, and receives lecture honoraria for Mead Johnson; is on the Advisory Board for Medela; and receives lecture honoraria from Abbott and Nestle.

Caroline Signore, MD, MPH (Guest Editor) has stock/ownership in Thoratec.

Disclosure of Discussion of Non-FDA Approved Uses for Pharmaceutical Products and/or Medical Devices.

The University of Virginia School of Medicine, as an ACCME provider, requires that all faculty presenters identify and disclose any off-label uses for pharmaceutical and medical device products. The University of Virginia School of Medicine recommends that each physician fully review all the available data on new products or procedures prior to clinical use.

TO ENROLL

To enroll in the Clinics in Perinatology Continuing Medical Education program, call customer service at 1-800-654-2452 or visit us online at www.theclinics.com/home/cme. The CME program is available to subscribers for an additional fee of $196.00.

THE CLINICS ARE NOW AVAILABLE ONLINE!

Access your subscription at:
www.theclinics.com

Foreword
The Tug of War between Vaginal and Cesarean Births

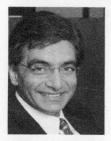

Lucky Jain, MD, MBA
Consulting Editor

It is hard to believe that in this day and age of nanomedicine,[1] regenerative medicine,[2] and other major medical advances, we are still debating the best way to deliver a baby! In fact, this debate has recently escalated due largely to a rapid rise in cesarean sections worldwide.[3] The issue is arguably complex, with multiple competing interests and considerations. There is also the overlay of risk tolerance, as parents and clinicians struggle to balance the risk of transient but commonly seen complications, with the rare chance of a catastrophic event.

Vaginal birth after a previous cesarean (VBAC) section exemplifies this dilemma. After years of trying to increase the number of VBAC deliveries, many hospitals had all but given up on this practice, unable to meet the requirements for anesthesia coverage and general preparedness for an emergency cesarean section in the event of failed trial of labor. Meanwhile, as primary and repeat cesarean section rates continue to rise, scientists are sorting through the published literature to come up with meaningful recommendations to reverse these trends. The recent NICHD workshop on Trial of Labor after Previous Cesarean is an example of such an effort.[4] We are pleased that this issue of *Clinics in Perinatology* is devoted to this important topic. Drs Landon and Signore are to be congratulated for the superb set of articles in this issue. These articles highlight the challenges faced by practitioners and opportunities for revisiting VBAC without increasing the risk to the mother or her fetus. It will remain to be seen if this renewed focus on VBACs will have a desired effect on cesarean section rates; it is also not clear if a broad set of recommendations can be applied to hospitals and providers in diverse settings. This discussion, however, does set the stage for new research into comparative effectiveness of various approaches.

Clin Perinatol 38 (2011) xiii–xiv
doi:10.1016/j.clp.2011.03.013
0095-5108/11/$ – see front matter © 2011 Elsevier Inc. All rights reserved.

I am particularly thankful to Kerry Holland at Elsevier for committing an issue of the *Clinics* to this important topic and to the authors and editors for their superb contributions.

Lucky Jain, MD, MBA
Department of Pediatrics
Emory University School of Medicine
2015 Uppergate Drive
Atlanta, GA 30322, USA

E-mail address:
ljain@emory.edu

REFERENCES

1. Kim BY, Rutka JT, Chan WC. Nanomedicine. N Engl J Med 2010;363(25):2434–43.
2. Jopling C, Boue S, Izpisua Belmonte JC. Dedifferentiation, transdifferentiation and reprogramming: three routes to regeneration. Nat Rev Mol Cell Biol 2011;12(2): 79–89.
3. Martin JA, Hamilton BE, Sutton PD, et al. Births: final data for 2007. Natl Vital Stat Rep 2010;58(24):1–85.
4. Signore C, Spong CY. Vaginal birth after cesarean: new insights manuscripts from an NIH Consensus Development Conference. March 8–10, 2010. Semin Perinatol 2010;34(5):309–10.

Preface

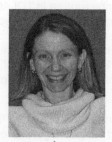 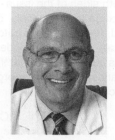

Caroline Signore, MD, MPH   Mark B. Landon, MD
Guest Editors

Cesarean delivery rates in the United States have now reached their highest levels ever, accounting for almost one third of all births. The inexorable rise in cesarean deliveries, especially in the last 15 years, has been fueled by a steady increase in primary cesareans and a sharp and persistent decrease in vaginal birth after cesarean (VBAC). The precise reasons behind these two trends are not entirely clear, but most agree that that multiple medical and societal forces are impacting choices for route of delivery. One thing remains certain, however: as long as these two individual trends continue, total cesarean delivery rates will continue to increase.

The appropriate utilization of trial of labor after cesarean (TOLAC)/VBAC has been a topic of much interest and debate among maternity caregivers, women, and other stakeholders in recent years. A key contributor to the controversy is the juxtaposition of maternal and fetal risks: cesarean delivery, especially multiple repeat cesareans, are widely recognized as carrying greater risk for maternal morbidity and mortality as compared to successful VBAC. On the other hand, catastrophic fetal outcomes—although rare in absolute terms—are more common in attempted VBAC than in scheduled repeat cesarean delivery. A troubling development in the care for women with previous cesarean has been the evolution and growth of restrictive practices and policies that limit women's access to TOLAC/VBAC.

It was with these concerns in mind that the National Institutes of Health held a Consensus Development Conference in March, 2010, to examine the evidence on maternal and neonatal outcomes, as well as the complex constellation of other factors affecting VBAC utilization, and to reach evidence-based consensus on the appropriate place for VBAC as a childbirth option. At the conclusion of the two and a half day conference, an objective panel of experts issued its consensus statement, affirming that a trial of labor remains a reasonable option for many women with a prior cesarean delivery and that access to TOLAC/VBAC requires additional attention.

In this issue of *Clinics in Perinatology*, our goal has been to present to a wide audience a thorough consideration of the issues facing clinicians and women contemplating delivery after prior cesarean. First, data on trends and patterns of VBAC utilization and access are presented. A number of articles then examine the multiple health system and ethical issues that impact the availability and use of TOLAC and

Clin Perinatol 38 (2011) xv–xvi
doi:10.1016/j.clp.2011.03.014   **perinatology.theclinics.com**
0095-5108/11/$ – see front matter © 2011 Elsevier Inc. All rights reserved.

VBAC. VBAC success rates are discussed, along with care practices that obstetricians and midwives employ that influence success rates and various outcomes. The serious potential complications on both sides of the issue—uterine rupture in TOLAC and disorders of placental implantation with multiple cesareans—are reviewed. Finally, short- and long-term maternal, fetal, and child outcomes are examined.

It is our hope that readers will gain insight and understanding of the complex medical issue of delivery after previous cesarean and that these insights will be helpful to practitioners, women, and health care institutions and organizations as they engage in dialogue and decision-making concerning this issue.

Caroline Signore, MD, MPH
Pregnancy and Perinatology Branch
Eunice Kennedy Shriver National Institute of
Child Health and Human Development
Bethesda, MD 20892, USA

Mark B. Landon, MD
Division of Maternal Fetal Medicine
Department of Obstetrics and Gynecology
Ohio State University College of Medicine
Columbus, OH 43210, USA

E-mail addresses:
signorec@mail.nih.gov (C. Signore)
mark.landon@osumc.edu (M.B. Landon)

Recent Trends and Patterns in Cesarean and Vaginal Birth After Cesarean (VBAC) Deliveries in the United States

Marian MacDorman, PhD[a],*, Eugene Declercq, PhD[b],
Fay Menacker, DrPH, CPNP[c]

KEYWORDS

- Cesarean delivery • Primary cesarean
- Vaginal birth after cesarean • VBAC • United States
- International comparisons

In 2008, approximately 1.4 million women in the United States had a cesarean delivery, representing 32.3% of all births.[1] Cesarean delivery continues to be the most common major surgical procedure for women in the United States.[2] In addition, because of increases in primary cesarean delivery, an increasing number of US women approach birth having already had at least 1 previous cesarean delivery.[3] This article examines the trends and patterns in total, primary, and repeat cesarean deliveries, in vaginal birth after cesarean (VBAC), and in the percentage of women who have had a prior cesarean.

METHODS

Data on the method of delivery used in this article are as reported on the more than 4 million birth certificates filed each year in the United States and compiled by the National Center for Health Statistics. Data on cesarean delivery became available from birth certificates in 1989, and by 1991, all US states were reporting this information.

Financial disclosure and conflict of interest: The authors have nothing to disclose.
[a] Division of Vital Statistics, Reproductive Statistics Branch, National Center for Health Statistics, Centers for Disease Control and Prevention, 3311 Toledo Road, Room 7318, Hyattsville, MD 20782, USA
[b] Department of Community Health Sciences, Boston University School of Public Health, 715 Albany Street, Boston, MA 02118, USA
[c] Social & Scientific Systems, Inc, 8757 Georgia Avenue, 12th Floor, Silver Spring, MD 20910, USA
* Corresponding author.
E-mail address: mfm1@cdc.gov

Clin Perinatol 38 (2011) 179–192
doi:10.1016/j.clp.2011.03.007
0095-5108/11/$ – see front matter. Published by Elsevier Inc.

(All states but Oklahoma reported this information in 1990.) Before 1989, data from the National Hospital Discharge Survey were used to track the trends in cesarean delivery.[4] The 2008 preliminary birth data (summary statistics)[1] and the 2007 final birth data (detailed characteristics)[3] were the latest data available at the time of manuscript preparation.

Revision of the US Standard Certificate of Live Birth

Beginning in 2003, some states began adopting the 2003 revision of the US Standard Certificate of Live Birth (revised). Although both revised and unrevised birth certificates contain information on the method of delivery, the format and wording of the method of delivery item is different between revised and unrevised birth certificates. Data on total cesarean delivery is comparable between the 2 revisions and is available for the United States as a whole throughout the period.[3,5–7] However, data on whether a woman has had a prior cesarean delivery is not comparable between the 2 revisions, which has the potential to affect several cesarean delivery measures.[3,6,7]

For 2003 and 2004 data, only a few states had revised their birth certificates, and national estimates on VBAC and primary and repeat cesarean deliveries were produced based primarily on unrevised birth certificate data.[5] However, beginning with 2005 data, it is not possible to produce comparable national estimates for primary and repeat cesarean deliveries, and VBAC rates and thus subnational estimates must be used.[3,6,7] For example, in 2007, revised data on VBAC and primary and repeat cesarean deliveries are available for 22 states, representing 53% of US births, including California, Colorado, Delaware, Florida, Idaho, Indiana, Iowa, Kansas, Kentucky, Nebraska, New Hampshire New York State (excluding New York City), North Dakota, Ohio, Pennsylvania, South Carolina, South Dakota, Tennessee, Texas, Vermont, Washington, and Wyoming.[3] Results for this 22-state area are not generalizable to the United States as a whole because they are not a random sample of all births. In particular, Mexican women are overrepresented in these data, whereas non-Hispanic white and non-Hispanic black women are underrepresented.[8] Therefore the trend data on US VBAC rates presented in **Fig. 1** ends in 2004.

Computation of Measures and Analytic Methods

Cesarean delivery measures are computed as shown in **Table 1**. Briefly, the total cesarean rate is the percentage of cesarean births out of all births in a given year. The primary cesarean rate is the percentage of cesarean births to women who have not had a previous cesarean delivery. The repeat cesarean rate is the percentage of cesarean births to women who have had a previous cesarean delivery. The rate of VBAC is the complement of the repeat cesarean rate and is the percentage of vaginal births to women who have had a previous cesarean delivery. Another important measure is the percentage of women with a prior cesarean delivery, which is the number of births to women with a prior cesarean delivery divided by the total number of live births. This measure represents the population of women who are eligible for either a repeat cesarean delivery or a VBAC. This measure may be computed for the total population or for women with at least 1 prior live birth.

The various cesarean delivery measures were analyzed by maternal age, maternal race/ethnicity, maternal education, birthplace of the mother, live birth order (number of previous live births plus the index birth), plurality, trimester of pregnancy when prenatal care began, and state. VBAC rates were also calculated by the number of prior cesarean deliveries.

For the birth attendant and place of delivery variables, the percentage of VBACs per 100 total births was computed. This measure indicates the prevalence of VBACs

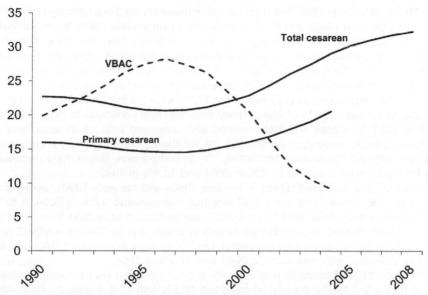

Fig. 1. US total cesarean rate 1990–2008 and the primary cesarean and VBAC rates 1990–2004. (*Data from* the National Vital Statistics System, Natality Data File.)

among women giving birth. This alternative measure is used because the standard denominator for VBAC rates (VBACs + repeat cesarean deliveries) is not useful for the measurement of midwife-attended births or home births because cesarean deliveries performed by midwives nor do they occur at home.

RESULTS
Trends

In 2008, nearly one-third (32.3%) of US babies were delivered by cesarean, the highest rate ever reported in the United States.[1] The total cesarean rate has increased by 56%

Table 1			
Computation of cesarean measures			
Total cesarean rate	$\dfrac{\text{Total number of births by cesarean}}{\text{Total number of births}} \times 100$		
Primary cesarean rate	$\dfrac{\text{Number of cesarean births to women with no previous cesarean delivery}}{\text{Number of primary cesarean births + number of vaginal births (not VBACs)}} \times 100$		
Repeat cesarean rate	$\dfrac{\text{Number of cesarean births to women with a previous cesarean delivery}}{\text{Number of VBACs + number of repeat cesarean births}} \times 100$		
VBAC rate	$\dfrac{\text{Number of vaginal births to women with a previous cesarean delivery}}{\text{Number of VBACs + number of repeat cesarean births}} \times 100$		
Percentage of women with a prior cesarean delivery	$\dfrac{\text{Number of births to women who had a prior cesarean delivery}}{\text{Total number of births}} \times 100$		

from 20.7% of births in 1996. The total cesarean rate increased dramatically during the 1970s and the early 1980s and then began to decline in the late 1980s (based on data from the National Hospital Discharge Survey).[4,9] Between 1990 and 1996, the total cesarean rate decreased as a result of a decrease in the primary cesarean rate and an increase in the VBAC rate (see **Fig. 1**).[3,5–7,9] Since 1996, these trends have reversed, and both primary and repeat cesarean rates have increased over the past decade.[1,3]

The primary cesarean rate increased from 14.6% of births in 1996 to 20.6% of births in 2004, an increase of 41%.[5] The primary cesarean rate continued to increase from 2004 to 2007 for states with both revised and unrevised birth certificates, and in 2007, the primary cesarean rate was 23.4% for the 22-state reporting area (states that had adopted the revised certificate).[3,6,7] In comparison, the primary cesarean rate for the 22-state area was 21.1% in 2004 and 14.5% in 1996.

The VBAC rate increased rapidly in the late 1980s and the early 1990s, peaking at 28.3% in 1996. Since 1996, the VBAC rate has decreased to 9.2% in 2004, a 67% decline from the peak in 1996.[5] The VBAC rate continued to decline from 2004 to 2007 for both revised and unrevised reporting areas, and in 2007, the VBAC rate was 8.3% for the 22-state area revised states.[3,6,7] In comparison, the VBAC rate for the same 22-state area was 8.6% in 2004 and 27.3% in 1996.

The percentage of births to mothers with a prior cesarean delivery was relatively stable during the 1990s, fluctuating between 10.5% and 10.8% (**Fig. 2**). Beginning in 1999, the percentage of births to mothers with a prior cesarean delivery increased from 10.6% births in 1999 to 12.1% in 2004, a 14% increase. This percentage continued to increase from 2004 to 2007 for both revised and unrevised states. In 2007, the percentage of births to women with a prior cesarean delivery was 12.9% for the 22-state reporting area (**Table 2**), compared with 12.0% in 2004 and 10.8% in 1996 for the same 22-state area. The total percentage of births to women with a prior cesarean delivery is useful for illustrating the effect of prior cesarean delivery on a population as a whole. However, a more precise indicator of the population at risk of having had a prior cesarean delivery is women who have had a prior live birth. In

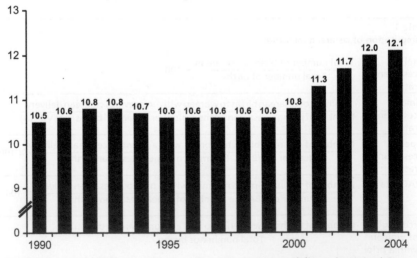

Fig. 2. Percentage of births to women with a prior cesarean delivery in United States for 1990–2004. (*Data from* the National Vital Statistics System, Natality Data File.)

2007, 21.3% of women with a prior live birth in the 22-state area had had a previous cesarean delivery.

Cross-Sectional Analysis of 2007 Data from 22 States

Table 2 presents total and primary cesarean rates, VBAC rates, and the percentage of births to women with a prior cesarean delivery by selected characteristics for the 22 revised states, representing 53% of US births. The total cesarean rate for the 22-state area was 32.3%, just 1% higher than the rate for the United States as a whole in 2007 (31.8%). Although the 22-state area is not representative of the United States as a whole, total cesarean rates by the characteristics shown in **Table 2** were quite similar between the 22-state area and the United States as a whole (data not shown).

Maternal age
The total and primary cesarean rates and the percentage of births to women with a prior cesarean delivery increased with increasing maternal age. Nearly one-fourth (23.1%) of teenaged mothers had a cesarean delivery, compared with nearly half (47.2%) of mothers aged 40 to 44 years and more than half (58.4%) of mothers 45 years and older. The primary cesarean rate for teenaged mothers was 21.0, compared with a rate of 49.3 for mothers 45 years and older. The percentage of births to women with a prior cesarean delivery increased from 3.1% for teenaged mothers to 21.8% for mothers aged 40 to 44 years. About 20.4% of mothers aged 45 years and older had had a prior cesarean delivery. In contrast, the VBAC rate showed little systematic pattern by maternal age. The VBAC rate varied from 7.5% to 8.5% for all age groups, except for women aged 45 years and older who had a lower VBAC rate (5.9%).

Maternal race/ethnicity
The variation in cesarean rates by maternal race/ethnicity was much smaller than the variation by maternal age. The total cesarean rate was lower than the national average for American Indian (29.2), Mexican (30.7), and Asian or Pacific Islander (31.9) mothers, close to the national average for non-Hispanic white (32.1) mothers and higher than the national average for Central or South American (33.2), Puerto Rican (33.9), and non-Hispanic black (34.3) mothers. For Cuban mothers, the total cesarean rate was 50.8, the highest rate among the race and ethnic groups, due mostly to a high primary cesarean rate (43.0). In general, patterns for the primary cesarean rates mirrored those for the total cesarean rate.

The VBAC rate was lowest for Cuban (2.0) and Central or South American (6.3) women and highest for non-Hispanic black (9.9) and American Indian (10.0) women.

The percentage of births to women with a prior cesarean delivery was lowest for Asian or Pacific Islander (12.0) and non-Hispanic white (12.1) women and highest for Mexican (14.8) and Cuban (14.2) women.

Maternal education
Both total and primary cesarean rates were highest for women who had attended college and lowest for women with less than a high-school diploma. In contrast, the VBAC rates were highest for women with less than a high-school diploma (9.1%) and lowest for women who had attended college (7.9%). There was little variation in the percentage of births to women with a prior cesarean delivery by maternal education.

Birthplace of the mother
There was little variation in the total cesarean rate by the birthplace of the mother. However, the primary cesarean rates were higher for mothers born in the 50 states

Table 2
Total and primary cesarean rates, VBAC rates, and percentage of births to women with a prior cesarean delivery by selected characteristics in 22 states in 2007

	Total Cesarean Rate[a]	Primary Cesarean Rate[b]	VBAC Rate[c]	Percentage of Births to Women with a Prior Cesarean Delivery[d]
Total	32.2	23.4	8.3	12.9
Maternal age				
<20 y	23.1	21.0	8.4	3.1
20–24 y	27.9	21.0	7.5	9.6
25–29 y	31.1	22.2	8.7	12.9
30–34 y	36.1	24.9	8.5	16.7
35–39 y	42.4	29.4	8.0	20.7
40–44 y	47.2	34.9	8.3	21.8
>45 y	58.4	49.3	5.9	20.4
Maternal race/ethnicity				
Non-Hispanic white	32.1	23.9	8.4	12.1
Non-Hispanic black	34.3	25.6	9.9	13.5
American Indian	29.2	20.1	10.0	13.0
Asian or Pacific Islander	31.9	23.8	8.0	12.0
All Hispanics[e]	31.8	21.6	7.4	14.4
Mexican	30.7	20.0	7.8	14.8
Puerto Rican	33.9	24.9	8.2	13.5
Cuban	50.8	43.0	2.0	14.2
Central or South American	33.2	24.2	6.3	12.9
Maternal education				
Less than high-school graduate	28.5	19.1	9.1	13.0
High-school graduate or GED completed	31.2	22.3	8.2	12.8
Some college	34.6	26.0	7.9	13.0
Birthplace of the mother				
Born in the 50 states and Washington, DC	32.3	23.9	8.1	12.4
Born outside the 50 states and Washington, DC	32.2	22.1	8.4	14.5
Live birth order				
1	31.9	31.8	n/a	n/a
2	34.0	17.1	6.1	22.0
3	32.1	15.5	8.3	21.8
4	29.7	15.2	12.5	20.1
5+	27.4	15.2	18.9	18.6
Plurality				
Single	30.8	21.8	8.5	12.9
Twin	75.4	71.7	2.9	14.6
Triplet/+	94.6	94.1	1.5	12.4

(continued on next page)

	Total Cesarean Rate[a]	Primary Cesarean Rate[b]	VBAC Rate[c]	Percentage of Births to Women with a Prior Cesarean Delivery[d]
Trimester when prenatal care began				
First	33.5	24.5	7.3	13.2
Second	29.7	21.1	9.9	12.4
Third	28.3	19.5	11.6	12.7
No prenatal care	26.7	20.5	18.3	10.4

Table 2
(continued)

Abbreviation: GED, general educational development.
[a] Number of cesareans per 100 total births; see **Table 1** for definitions.
[b] Number of primary cesareans per 100 births to women with no prior cesarean delivery.
[c] Number of VBACs per 100 women who had a prior cesarean delivery.
[d] Number of births to women with a prior cesarean delivery per 100 total births.
[e] Includes other Hispanic origin and unknown Hispanic origin not shown separately.
Data from the National Vital Statistics System, Natality Data File.

and Washington, DC (23.9), compared with mothers born outside the 50 states and Washington, DC (22.1). In contrast, the VBAC rates were slightly lower for mothers born in the 50 states and Washington, DC (8.1%), compared with mothers born elsewhere (8.4%). A lower percentage of mothers born in the 50 states and Washington, DC had had a prior cesarean delivery (12.4%), compared with mothers born elsewhere (14.5%).

Live birth order
About 31.9% of mothers having their first live birth had a cesarean delivery. Cesarean rates were highest (34.0) for mothers having their second live birth and then gradually declined for mothers having their third (32.1), fourth (29.7), or fifth or greater (27.4) live birth.

Compared with mothers having their first live birth, primary cesarean rates were 46% lower for mothers who had successfully had 1 prior vaginal delivery (17.1), and declined further for women who had had 2 (15.5) or 3 or more (15.2) prior vaginal deliveries (see **Table 2**). In contrast, the VBAC rates were lowest (6.1%) for women having their second live birth, but increased sharply with increasing birth order. For example, compared with women having their second live birth, the VBAC rate was double for women having their fourth live birth (12.5) and triple for women having their fifth or higher order live birth (18.9). The percentage of births to women with a prior cesarean delivery was highest for women having their second live birth (22.0%) and declined thereafter with increasing live birth order.

Plurality
Cesarean rates were higher for multiple births than for single births. About 30.8% of single births were cesarean deliveries, compared with 75.4% for twins and 94.6% for triplet or higher order births. Primary cesarean rates followed a similar pattern. The VBAC rates were lower for women with multiple pregnancies, 8.5% for singletons, compared with 2.9% for twins and 1.5% for triplet or higher-order pregnancies.

Trimester of pregnancy when prenatal care began
Total cesarean rates were higher for women who began prenatal care in the first trimester of pregnancy (33.5) and lowest for women with no prenatal care (26.7).

Patterns were similar for primary cesarean rates. Women who began prenatal care in the first trimester were more likely to have had a prior cesarean (13.2%) compared with women beginning care in the second (12.4%) or third (12.7%) trimester or those with no prenatal care (10.4%). In contrast, the VBAC rates were lowest for women who began prenatal care in the first trimester of pregnancy (7.3) and increased for women beginning care in the second (9.9) or third (11.6) trimester or those with no prenatal care (18.3).

Number of prior cesarean deliveries
VBAC rates declined as the number of previous cesarean deliveries increased. The VBAC rate was 10.1% for women with 1 prior cesarean delivery compared with 3.2% for women with 2 prior cesarean deliveries and 2.8% for women with 3 or more prior cesarean deliveries (**Fig. 3**).

Place of delivery and birth attendant
The percentage of total births that were VBACs was higher for home births than for hospital births. In 2007, in the 22-state area, 3.6% of home births were VBACs compared with 1.6% of birthing center births and 1.0% of hospital births. Home births comprised 0.7% of all live births and 2.2% of VBACs. Patterns were similar when data were examined by birth attendant. In 2007, for the 22-state area, 1.4% of births attended by certified nurse midwives were VBACs compared with 2.5% of births attended by other midwives and 1.0% of births attended by physicians.

State
There were large differences in the various cesarean delivery measures by state for the 22 states reporting revised method of delivery data in 2007 (**Table 3**). Total cesarean rates varied from a low of 23.8% for Idaho to a high of 37.2% for Florida, and primary cesarean rates varied from a low of 16.3% for Idaho to a high of 28.6% for Florida. VBAC rates varied from a low of 4.7% for California to a high of 19.4% for Vermont. The percentage of births to women with a prior cesarean delivery varied from a low of 9.3% in Colorado and New Hampshire to a high of 15.6% in New York State (excluding New York City).

For 13 of the 22 states, lower-than-average total and primary cesarean rates were associated with higher VBAC rates and a lower percentage of births to women with a prior cesarean (Colorado, Idaho, Indiana, Iowa, Kansas, New Hampshire, North Dakota, Ohio, Pennsylvania, South Dakota, Vermont, Washington, and Wyoming). In contrast, in Florida and New York State (excluding New York City), higher total and primary cesarean rates were associated with lower VBAC rates and a higher

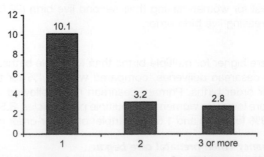

Fig. 3. VBAC rate by number of previous cesareans for 22 states in 2007. *(Data from* the National Vital Statistics System, Natality Data File.)

Table 3
Total and primary cesarean rates, VBAC rates, and percentage of births to women with a prior cesarean delivery by state for 22 revised states for 2007

State	Total Cesarean Rate	Primary Cesarean Rate	VBAC Rate	Percentage of Births with a Prior Cesarean
Total	32.2	23.4	8.3	12.9
California	32.1	21.4	4.7	14.4
Colorado	25.8	19.9	16.2	9.3
Delaware	31.9	21.3	9.8	15.3
Florida	37.2	28.6	5.5	13.0
Idaho	23.8	16.3	14.3	10.7
Indiana	29.3	22.4	9.7	10.2
Iowa	29.4	21.3	9.3	11.7
Kansas	29.8	21.4	9.6	12.2
Kentucky	34.6	26.3	5.7	12.3
Nebraska	30.9	21.5	7.9	13.3
New Hampshire	29.5	23.6	12.7	9.3
New York State (excluding New York City)	35.5	24.9	7.4	15.6
North Dakota	28.3	19.9	10.6	12.1
Ohio	29.8	22.0	12.4	11.9
Pennsylvania	30.0	22.3	13.8	11.9
South Carolina	33.4	25.1	10.0	12.7
South Dakota	26.6	18.4	14.2	12.3
Tennessee	33.3	25.4	9.5	12.1
Texas	33.7	25.0	9.3	13.3
Vermont	26.9	19.6	19.4	12.0
Washington	28.9	22.0	12.6	10.5
Wyoming	26.6	18.2	8.7	11.5

Data from the National Vital Statistics System, Natality Data File.

percentage of births to women with a prior cesarean delivery. Other states showed a mixed pattern (California, Delaware, Kentucky, Nebraska, South Carolina, Tennessee, and Texas).

International Comparisons

Among 26 industrialized countries that provided data to the Organization for Economic Cooperation and Development, cesarean rates ranged from a low of 14% for the Netherlands to a high of 40% for Italy in 2007 (**Fig. 4**).[10] The total cesarean rate in the United States (32%) was higher than the rate for 22 countries. Only 3 countries had rates that were higher than the US rate. When compared with the US rate, the Canadian rate was 16% lower, the rate for the United Kingdom was 25% lower, the French rate was 38% lower, and the Dutch rate was 56% lower.

VBAC rates for selected industrialized countries in 2004 are shown in **Fig. 5**. These data were largely drawn from the European Perinatal Health Report,[3,11,12] and VBAC data were not available for many of the countries that reported information on total cesarean rates (see **Fig. 4**). The US has the lowest VBAC rate among the 14

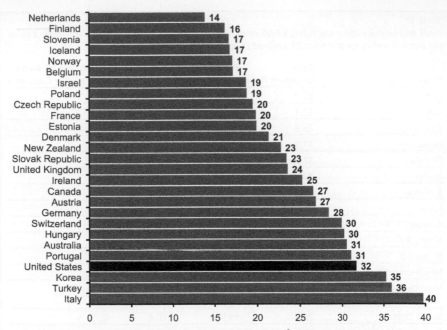

Fig. 4. Total cesarean rate for selected industrialized countries in 2007. (*Data from* Organization for Economic Cooperation and Development. OECD health data. 2010. Available at: http://www.ecosante.org/index2.php?base5OCDE&langh5ENG&langs5ENG&sessionid. Accessed October 25, 2010.)

industrialized countries. In fact, the US VBAC rate is less than half the rate for the next lowest country (Lithuania). The VBAC rate for France is nearly 4 times the US rate, the rate for Germany is 4.5 times the US rate, the rate for Sweden is 5 times the US rate, and the rate for the Netherlands, the country with the highest VBAC rate, is more than

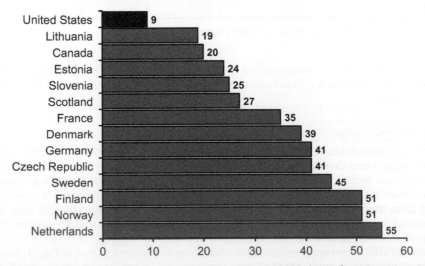

Fig. 5. VBAC rates for selected industrialized countries in 2004. (*Data from* European Perinatal Health Report for European data, Statistics Canada for Canadian data, National Center for Health Statistics for US data.)

6 times the US rate. In fact, in the Netherlands, Norway, and Finland, more than half of births to women with a prior cesarean delivery are VBACs.

DISCUSSION

The total cesarean rate increased by 56% from 20.7% of births in 1996 to nearly one-third (32.3%) of US births in 2008, the highest rate ever recorded in the United States.[1,3] The recent increase in the total cesarean rate is because of both an increase in the primary cesarean rate and a decrease in the VBAC rate. In 2007, only 8.3% of women with a prior cesarean delivery had a VBAC in a 22-state area. Thus, a first cesarean delivery now virtually guarantees that subsequent deliveries will be cesarean deliveries. As both primary and repeat cesarean deliveries have become more common, the percentage of women with a prior cesarean delivery has also increased. In 2007 21.3% of women with a prior live birth had had a previous cesarean delivery in a 22-state area, which suggests that further increases in the cesarean rate are likely.

Strengths of the birth certificate data to track trends in cesarean delivery include the comprehensive population-based nature of these data, which include all births in the United States for a given year. Most demographic items and some medical items (including live birth order and method of delivery) are considered to be well reported.[13,14] A major limitation of the study is the lack of comparability of the item on previous cesarean delivery between the unrevised and revised birth certificate data. Because of this limitation, data on primary cesarean, VBAC, and percentage of prior cesarean births are not available for the United States as a whole after 2004. Instead, the 2007 data for these variables were examined for the 22 states (representing 53% of US births) that had revised their birth certificates as of January 1, 2007. Although this 22-state area is not representative of the United States as a whole, it contains states from all regions of the country, and total cesarean rates by characteristics are similar to those for the United States as a whole.

Cesarean trends as a whole may have been influenced by the changes in practice guidelines and by the publication of key articles in major research journals. However, these factors have had a greater influence on the VBAC rates, which increased from 1989 to 1996, and then declined from 1996 onwards, thus representing 2 major shifts in the practice of American obstetrics within a relatively short period. **Fig. 6** illustrates the VBAC trends by month and the timing of notable publications. A series of studies by Flamm and colleagues[15,16] in the 1980s provided some of the early support for attempting trials of labor for women with repeat cesareans and the American College of Obstetricians and Gynecologists (ACOG)–issued guidelines encouraging VBAC in the 1980s likely contributing to the rising rate seen in the early 1990s.[17]

The major shift in trend occurred in 1996 following the publication of an article in the *New England Journal of Medicine* by McMahon and colleagues[18] that found higher rates of hysterectomy and uterine rupture in the trial of labor group compared with elective repeat cesarean in their Nova Scotia database. In October 1998, the ACOG issued new guidelines on VBAC that included a section based on level C evidence (expert opinion) calling for VBACs only "…in institutions equipped to respond to emergencies with physicians readily available."[19] After 9 months, in July 1999, the ACOG reissued the VBAC guidelines changing the word "readily," to "immediately,"[20] and the word "immediately" is still used in an August 2010 reissue of the guidelines, although with some qualifications.[21] In July 2001, an article was published on the use of induction in trials of labor, accompanied by an editorial that concluded that elective repeat cesareans were "unequivocally" safer for infants.[22,23] This article and editorial received widespread publicity and seemed to have an effect on the US

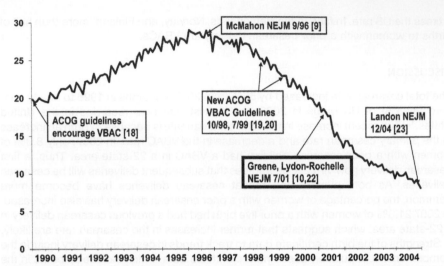

Fig. 6. VBAC rate by month, United States, 1990–2004. (*Data from* the National Vital Statistics System, Natality Data File.)

VBAC rates. In June 2001, the month before their publication, the national VBAC rate was 17.6%. By August 2001, the rate was down to 14.9%, a 15% decline in only 2 months, and by December, it had fallen to 13.4%, a 24% drop in 6 months.

In December 2004, a study by Landon and colleagues,[24] the largest multicenter study of trial of labor compared with elective cesarean, was published in the *New England Journal of Medicine*. The investigator found low rates of symptomatic uterine rupture (0.7%), fewer differences between outcomes, and low absolute risks for poor outcomes associated with VBACs. Although national data on VBAC rates have not been reported since 2004, there seems to be little evidence that the article by Landon and colleagues had any effect in terms of increasing or decreasing the VBAC rates.

Both total cesarean and VBAC rates varied by characteristics of the mother and the pregnancy. Cesarean rates were higher for older women, non-Hispanic black and Cuban women, women with some college education, women having multiple births, and women with early prenatal care. The VBAC rates were lower for Hispanic and Asian or Pacific Islander women, women aged 45 years and older, women having multiple births, women with early prenatal care, and women who attended college. The higher VBAC rates for women with late or no prenatal care suggest that not all VBACs are planned.

Although some researchers have expressed concerns about the safety of VBACs in a hospital setting,[18,23] in 2007, there were 540 home VBACs in the 22-state area. Of these VBACs, 394 were identified as planned home VBACs, 52 were unplanned, and for 94, the planning status was unknown. The number of home VBACs has been increasing in recent years among states with revised and unrevised birth certificates (data not shown). In 2003, 664 births in the United States as a whole were home VBACs. In 2007, VBACs comprised 3.9% of planned home births, compared with 1.0% of hospital births. It is possible that recent hospital policies limiting or prohibiting VBACs[25] have led some women to choose a home VBAC.

In 2007, the cesarean delivery rate ranged from a low of 14% in the Netherlands to a high of 40% in Italy. The US cesarean rate (32%) was higher than the rate for 22 countries but was lower than the rate for 3 countries. In 2004, the US VBAC rate (9%) was lowest among 14 industrialized countries; 3 countries had VBAC rates greater than 50%. In 1985, the World Health Organization stated that a cesarean rate of 15% may be reasonable for most populations.[26] Although controversy over the ideal level continues,[27] a recent international study found a decrease in maternal mortality associated with increases in cesarean rates of up to 15%. However, for countries with cesarean rates greater than 15%, higher cesarean rates were correlated with higher maternal mortality rates.[28] A second study for Latin America found similar results.[29] These data add to the increasing body of research on trends in method of delivery both in the United States and in other countries. Given the low rate of VBAC delivery, these data suggest that a woman who has a first cesarean delivery in the United States is unlikely to have a subsequent vaginal delivery.

REFERENCES

1. Hamilton BE, Martin JA, Ventura SJ. Births: preliminary data for 2008. National vital statistics reports, vol. 58. Hyattsville (MD): National Center for Health Statistics; 2010.
2. Hall MJ, DeFrances CJ, Williams SN, et al. National hospital discharge survey: 2007 summary. National health statistics reports no. 29. Hyattsville (MD): National Center for Health Statistics; 2010.
3. Martin JA, Hamilton BE, Sutton PD, et al. Births, Final Data for 2007. National vital statistics reports, vol. 58. Hyattsville (MD): National Center for Health Statistics; 2010.
4. Taffel SM, Placek PJ, Moien M, et al. 1989 U.S. cesarean section rate steadies—VBAC rate rises to nearly one in five. Birth 1991;18:73–7.
5. Martin JA, Hamilton BE, Sutton PD, et al. Births, final data for 2004. National vital statistics reports, vol. 55. Hyattsville (MD): National Center for Health Statistics; 2006.
6. Martin JA, Hamilton BE, Sutton PD, et al. Births, final data for 2005. National vital statistics reports, vol. 56. Hyattsville (MD): National Center for Health Statistics; 2007.
7. Martin JA, Hamilton BE, Sutton PD, et al. Births, final data for 2006. National vital statistics reports, vol. 57. Hyattsville (MD): National Center for Health Statistics; 2009.
8. National Center for Health Statistics. User's guide to the 2007 natality public-use file. Hyattsville (MD): National Center for Health Statistics; 2010. Available at: ftp://ftp.cdc.gov/pub/Health_Statistics/NCHS/Dataset_Documentation/DVS/natality/UserGuide2007.pdf. Accessed October 25, 2010.
9. MacDorman MF, Menacker F, Declercq E. Cesarean birth in the United States: epidemiology, trends and outcomes. Clin Perinatol 2008;35:293–307.
10. Organization for Economic Cooperation and Development. OECD health data. 2010. Available at: http://www.ecosante.org/index2.php?base=OCDE&langh=ENG&langs=ENG&sessionid. Accessed October 25, 2010.
11. EURO-PERISTAT project, with SCPE, EUROCAT, EURONEOSTAT. European perinatal health report. 2008. Available at: http://www.europeristat.com. Accessed October 25, 2010.
12. Canadian perinatal health report, 2008 edition. Ottawa (Canada): Public Health Agency of Canada; 2008.
13. Roohan PJ, Josberger RE, Acar J, et al. Validation of birth certificate data in New York State. J Community Health 2003;28:335–46.

14. DiGiuseppe DL, Araon DC, Ranbom L, et al. Reliability of birth certificate data: a multi-hospital comparison to medical records information. Matern Child Health J 2002;6:169–79.
15. Flamm BL, Lim OW, Jones C, et al. Vaginal birth after cesarean section: results of a multicenter study. Am J Obstet Gynecol 1988;158(5):1079–84.
16. Flamm BL, Newman LA, Thomas SJ, et al. Vaginal birth after cesarean delivery: results of a 5-year multicenter collaborative study. Obstet Gynecol 1990;76: 750–4.
17. American College of Obstetricians and Gynecologists. Guidelines for vaginal delivery after previous cesarean birth. Washington, DC: The American College of Obstetricians and Gynecologists; 1988.
18. McMahon MJ, Luther ER, Bowes WA Jr, et al. Comparison of a trial of labor with an elective second cesarean section. N Engl J Med 1996;335(10):689–95.
19. American College of Obstetricians and Gynecologists. ACOG practice bulletin No. 2. Vaginal birth after previous cesarean delivery. Obstet Gynecol 1998; 92(3):1–7.
20. American College of Obstetricians and Gynecologists. ACOG practice bulletin No. 5. Vaginal birth after previous cesarean delivery. Obstet Gynecol 1999; 94(1):1–8.
21. American College of Obstetricians and Gynecologists. ACOG practice bulletin No. 115. Vaginal birth after previous cesarean delivery. Obstet Gynecol 2010; 116(2):450–63.
22. Lydon-Rochelle M, Holt VL, Easterling TR, et al. Risk of uterine rupture during labor among women with a prior cesarean delivery. N Engl J Med 2001;345(1): 3–8.
23. Greene MF. Vaginal delivery after cesarean section–is the risk acceptable? N Engl J Med 2001;345(1):54–5.
24. Landon MB, Hauth JC, Leveno KJ, et al. Maternal and perinatal outcomes associated with a trial of labor after prior cesarean delivery. N Engl J Med 2004; 351(25):2581–9.
25. National Institutes of Health. National Institutes of Health Consensus Development conference statement: vaginal birth after cesarean: new insights, March 8–10, 2010. Obstet Gynecol 2010;115:1279–95.
26. World Health Organization. Appropriate technology for birth. Lancet 1985;2: 436–7.
27. Resnik R. Can a 29% cesarean delivery rate possibly be justified? Obstet Gynecol 2006;107:752–3.
28. Betran AP, Merialdi M, Lauer JA, et al. Rates of caesarean section: analysis of global, regional and national estimates. Paediatr Perinat Epidemiol 2007;21: 98–113.
29. Villar J, Valladares E, Wojdyla D, et al. Caesarean delivery rates and pregnancy outcomes: the 2005 WHO global survey on maternal and perinatal health in Latin America. Lancet 2006;367(9525):1819–29.

Nonclinical Factors Affecting Women's Access to Trial of Labor After Cesarean Delivery

Lisa M. Korst, MD, PhD[a,b,*], Kimberly D. Gregory, MD, MPH[c,d,e],
Moshe Fridman, PhD[f], Jeffrey P. Phelan, MD, JD[g]

KEYWORDS

- Vaginal birth after cesarean • Cesarean • Medical liability
- Obstetric health services • Obstetric information systems

In March 2010, the National Institutes of Health (NIH) convened a Consensus Development Conference to advance understanding of both medical and nonmedical factors contributing to the rapidly falling rate of vaginal birth after cesarean (VBAC).[1] The rate of VBAC, defined as the proportion of women with prior cesarean delivery who deliver vaginally, steadily increased from 1989 (18.9%) to 1996 (28.3%), but has been decreasing each year since then, to 8.3% in 2007 (**Fig. 1**).[2] Gregory and colleagues[3] examined trends in trial of labor after cesarean (TOLAC) rates from data from the Nationwide Inpatient Sample (NIS) for the years 2000, 2003, and 2005, drawing on previously described methods for calculating these rates from

Dr Gregory is employed by Cedars-Sinai Medical Center. The remaining authors have nothing to disclose.

[a] Department of Obstetrics & Gynecology, Keck School of Medicine, University of Southern California, IRD Building, 2020 Zonal Avenue, #201, Los Angeles, CA 90033, USA
[b] Childbirth Research Associates, LLC, 12439 Magnolia Boulevard, #154, North Hollywood, CA 91607, USA
[c] Department of Obstetrics & Gynecology, Burns Allen Research Institute, Cedars-Sinai Medical Center, 8700 Beverly Boulevard, Suite 160 West, Los Angeles, CA 90048, USA
[d] Department of Obstetrics & Gynecology, David Geffen School of Medicine, 200 Medical Plaza, Suites 430 and 220, Los Angeles, CA 90095, USA
[e] Department of Community Health Sciences, UCLA School of Public Health, PO Box 951772, Los Angeles, CA 90095-1772, USA
[f] AMF Consulting, Inc, 846 South Citrus Avenue, Los Angeles, CA 90036, USA
[g] Department of Obstetrics and Gynecology, Citrus Valley Medical Center, 13181 Crossroads Parkway, North, Suite 380, City of Industry, West Covina, CA 91746, USA
* Corresponding author. Childbirth Research Associates, 12439 Magnolia Boulevard, #154, North Hollywood, CA 91607.
E-mail address: korst@usc.edu

Clin Perinatol 38 (2011) 193–216
doi:10.1016/j.clp.2011.03.004
0095-5108/11/$ – see front matter © 2011 Elsevier Inc. All rights reserved.

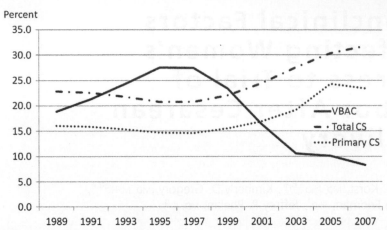

Fig. 1. Rates of total cesarean deliveries, primary cesarean deliveries, and VBAC, 1989 to 2007. (*Data from* the National Center for Health Statistics. NIH Consensus Development Conference on Vaginal Birth After Cesarean: New Insights; 2010. Bethesda (MD); with permission.)

administrative data.[4] The VBAC rate (as defined earlier), decreased from 28.2% to 13.8% to 10.3% across these years. Simultaneously, TOLAC rates (attempts/all priors) decreased from 40.9% to 21.5% to 17.0%, with VBAC success rates (VBAC/all attempts) decreasing less dramatically at 69.1%, 64.0%, and 60.3%.

These rate decreases associated with VBAC have been accompanied by a rapid increase in cesarean delivery (to 31.8% in 2007), and include increases in both primary and repeat cesareans.[2] Rate decreases are also evident for instrumental deliveries. At 4.3% in 2007, instrumental delivery reached its lowest rate ever, with use of forceps decreasing to 0.8% and vacuum extraction to 3.5%.[2] This compares with 1990, when approximately 1 in 20 infants was delivered with the assistance of forceps, and 1 in 25 delivered with vacuum assistance. Although data from the National Hospital Discharge Survey (NHDS) suggest that forceps and vacuum delivery may be underreported on the birth certificate, NHDS and birth certificate data have shown similar trends since 1990.[5]

In the intervening years since the first NIH conference on cesarean childbirth in 1981,[6] the risks to performing VBAC have not substantially changed: VBAC is successful 60% to 80% of the time, and it is associated with uterine rupture about 1% of the time.[7–9] After a succession of both independent and collaborative studies, and multiple meta-analyses, the absolute risks to both mother and fetus continue to seem to be low,[10] supporting the conference's conclusion that a trial of labor is a reasonable option for many pregnant women with 1 prior low, transverse uterine incision.[1]

The most recent Practice Bulletin from the American Congress of Obstetricians and Gynecologists (ACOG) regarding VBAC summarizes multiple studies in the last decade, comparing immediate maternal and neonatal morbidity and mortality from elective repeat cesarean delivery (ERCD) with trial of labor after 1 prior cesarean, and shows that, although all risks are low, the different delivery methods show a trade-off in risk for the mother versus the fetus. This trade-off makes the risk comparison difficult, as does the overall lack of ability to predict the future maternal consequences associated with complications of multiple cesarean deliveries such as hysterectomy, bowel or bladder injury, transfusion, infection, and abnormal placentation.

In a hypothetical cohort of 100,000 women, Guise and colleagues[11] summarized the numbers of maternal deaths, uterine ruptures, and perinatal deaths expected from

ERCD versus TOLAC, showing that ERCD is associated with slightly more maternal deaths, and TOLAC with more perinatal deaths (**Table 1**).

Table 1 suggests a 2.7-fold increased relative risk of perinatal deaths for TOLAC versus ERCD, but because of the low perinatal death probability, the number needed to treat is 1205 (95% confidence interval [CI] 906–1759), which is the number of ERCD required to prevent 1 perinatal death in a patient having TOLAC. For maternal deaths, the relative risk is 3.3 for ERCD versus TOLAC, but the number needed to treat is 11,111 (95% CI 5855–108,778), meaning that more than 10,000 trials of labor would be required to prevent 1 maternal death from ERCD.

Given the low absolute risks of TOLAC, the general consensus within the obstetric community is that attempting VBAC remains a safe option. In most cases, women with 1 previous cesarean delivery with a low, transverse incision are candidates for, and should be offered, a trial of labor. However, despite this well-established evidence and general consensus regarding risk, why do VBAC rates continue to decline? This disparity directs attention to the importance of a much wider societal or nonclinical context for VBAC, and it is within this context that potential causal factors for this decline must be explored, and potential solutions discovered. Guided by previous exhaustive work examining this societal context of VBAC,[12,13] this article considers 5 general categories of factors that seem to be influencing VBAC rates:

- Opinion leaders and professional guidelines
- Hospital facilities and cesarean availability
- Reimbursement for providing a trial of labor
- Medical liability
- Patient-level factors.

OPINION LEADERS AND GUIDELINES

There is some high-quality evidence that professional leadership in the obstetric community affects the use of cesarean and VBAC delivery. This influence seems to be operative at both local and national levels. In their systematic review, Kramer and colleagues[12] examined interventions designed to increase VBAC at the organizational level, and noted that the introduction of guidelines or policies to modify rates of delivery outcomes (typically to increase rates of TOLAC and VBAC) appeared effective. Lomas and colleagues[14] in 1991 also provided strong evidence that opinion leaders had a greater likelihood of changing practice compared with using audit and feedback. Two other studies,[15,16] completed before 1996, tracked VBAC rates and suggested that national guidelines did affect practice. After 1996, when the VBAC rate started to decline, there are scattered reports of continued efforts to promote VBAC, such as that of Misra[17] in 2008, who described a program to encourage VBAC in a Medicaid population.

Table 1		
Numbers of serious complications associated with TOLAC delivery versus ERCD in a hypothetical cohort of 100,0000 women, using statistically significant pooled risk estimates		
Outcome	TOLAC Delivery	ERCD
Maternal deaths	4	13
Uterine rupture	468	26
Perinatal deaths	133	50

Data from Guise JM, Denman MA, Emeis C, et al. Vaginal birth after cesarean: new insights on maternal and neonatal outcomes. Obstet Gynecol 2010;115(6):1276.

Anecdotally, there is a generally accepted historical description of events that appeared to influence VBAC rates. In 1980, in response to the tripling of the cesarean delivery rate from 5% to 16.5% in the previous decade, the NIH sponsored a conference on cesarean childbirth, and recommended that "in hospitals with appropriate facilities, services, and staff for prompt emergency cesarean birth, a proper selection of cases should permit a safe trial of labor and vaginal delivery for women who have had a previous low segment transverse cesarean birth."[6] They attributed 25% to 30% of the cesarean rate increase to repeat cesarean delivery, and looked to a growing body of literature documenting the relative safety of VBAC.

The most prominent concern regarding VBAC has always been the potential for the existing uterine scar to open, or rupture, during labor.[18] Such disruption may result in the disruption of the placenta, and cause fetal-maternal hemorrhage, which may lead to hypoxia, cardiovascular collapse, and brain injury or death in the fetus if not delivered promptly.[19] The incidence of uterine rupture in women with a prior scar is estimated to be slightly less than 1%,[13] but the immediacy of the response required, and the potential for permanent neurologic injury to the fetus, require caregivers to be extremely vigilant.

The publication of the NIH report encouraged extensive research activity regarding VBAC and, in the next decade, professional and public policy shifted to a wide acceptance of VBAC as a major component of strategies to avoid cesarean delivery.[20] In 1982, ACOG, responsible for setting national guidelines for the profession, issued its first publication on VBAC, acknowledging that, with careful selection of patients with previous low segment transverse uterine incisions and with proper facilities and staff, an attempt at vaginal delivery appeared to be an acceptable option.[21] According to Zinberg,[20] writing from his position as the Vice President of Practice Activities for ACOG, this guideline recommended that a "responsible physician who is capable of evaluating labor and performing a cesarean delivery should be in-house and immediately available to perform an emergency cesarean or to manage other complications." Further statements followed in 1984, 1988, 1994, 1995, and 1998, lessening the restrictions on patient eligibility and physician availability.[20]

VBAC rates rose rapidly, reaching a high of nearly 30% in 1996. The downward trend in VBAC began with the profession's growing awareness of VBAC-related morbidity and mortality, which was articulated in Phelan's[22] 1996 publication of an editorial in the popular *OBG Management* journal entitled, VBAC: time to reconsider? In that editorial, Phelan,[22] an early VBAC advocate and researcher, was the first to suggest a procedure-based consent form for VBAC candidates. This consent form contained the sentence: "I understand that if my uterus ruptures during my VBAC, there may not be sufficient time to operate and to prevent the death of or permanent brain injury to my baby." This sentence alone created a stir throughout the obstetric community, particularly because the consent form became widely favored by malpractice insurance carriers. The VBAC controversy was compounded by McMahon,[23] who emphasized the prevalence of complications of a failed VBAC. This was followed in 1998 by a Point/Counterpoint segment written by Flamm[24] and Phelan,[25] who presented opposing perspectives on the risks of VBAC. Although there was mutual agreement that the risk of uterine rupture during a VBAC was about 1%,[26] Phelan[25] emphasized that this risk was in addition to the usual risks associated with labor in patients without a uterine scar. By 1999, ACOG had adopted a more conservative position and required that a physician capable of monitoring labor and performing an emergency cesarean delivery be immediately available throughout active labor.[27] Within a short historical time frame, the VBAC trend rapidly reversed (see **Fig. 1**).

The use of the term immediately available generated much concern and confusion among ACOG members.[20,28] Since the mid-1980s, the standard for all emergency births had been the 30-minute rule, which, although not derived from an evidence base, was widely accepted as the upper limit on the cesarean decision to delivery interval.[29] According to Zinberg,[20] in addition to its concern for childbirth safety, ACOG sought to provide a defensible legal strategy for its members by requiring them to be present in the event of a VBAC complication. These guidelines were reiterated in a subsequent ACOG Practice Bulletin published in 2004,[30] and in the most recent Practice Bulletin from 2010.[10]

Although this immediate availability standard provided a defense in the event of a uterine rupture during a VBAC, it also created a separate class of patients and, at the same time, imposed a higher standard of care for patients having VBAC versus non-VBAC, suggesting a lesser standard of care for patients not having VBAC.

Furthermore, the immediate availability standard is likely only to prevent fetal brain injury or death when the patient's clinical signs and symptoms provide a warning or notice to the caregivers that the uterine rupture is occurring. The onset of the uterine rupture is identifiable in only about 50% of cases through the sudden appearance of moderate or severe variable decelerations at a time when they are not expected.[31] The appearance of these fetal heart rate decelerations constitutes a warning or notice that the uterine rupture is occurring. To estimate the number of cases of fetal neurologic injury that this standard is likely to prevent, it must be recognized that a fetus may experience fetal brain injury or death within as little as 18 minutes from the onset of the uterine rupture.[26] Catastrophic uterine ruptures, in which there is a partial or complete expulsion of the placenta and/or the fetus into the maternal abdomen, may have an even shorter window in which to prevent brain injury. Mobilizing resources within this brief window of opportunity is difficult, and depends on whether any warning occurred. Consequently, fetal brain injury in the circumstances of a catastrophic uterine rupture without warning would likely be nonpreventable. Given a uterine rupture rate of 1%, of which 50% occur without warning, and 25% are catastrophic,[26] approximately 1 in 800 VBACs would result in fetal brain injury that was still not prevented by the immediate availability standard. Although this risk is small, questions linger regarding whether the childbearing public remains willing to accept this risk, and whether third-party payers remain willing to reimburse hospitals and obstetricians for providing immediate availability.

Shihady and colleagues[32] and Roberts and colleagues[33] surveyed hospital administrators in a variety of states about clinical practices and policy changes after the 1999 ACOG recommendation. Both studies received response rates of more than 90%, and, in both series, approximately 30% of hospitals stated that they stopped allowing VBAC services. These non-VBAC hospitals largely cited the 1999 ACOG guideline and the importance of providing 24-hour availability of operating personnel as their rationale for not allowing VBAC. In the study by Roberts and colleagues,[33] of the hospitals that still allowed VBAC, 68% had to change their policies to be compliant with ACOG recommendations. The most frequent changes involved the in-house presence of surgery (53%) and anesthesia (44%) personnel when women desiring VBAC presented in labor. Compared with hospitals that stopped allowing VBAC, those that permitted VBAC were larger, closer to other delivery hospitals, annually delivered more babies, and annually had more cesarean deliveries. Gochnour and colleagues,[34] in a survey of physicians in Utah, reported that most were aware of ACOG recommendations, and 45% reported a decrease in their provision of VBAC. Physicians were less likely to report the capacity to immediately perform a cesarean in suburban and rural areas (100% urban, 88 suburban, and 76% rural), and physicians practicing in these areas reported the largest decline in the use of trial of labor.

This decrease in VBAC availability has elicited concern from quality-monitoring organizations such as the California Hospital Association and Reporting Task Force (CHART),[35] which has suggested that hospitals should be required to report whether they provide access to VBAC, a suggestion that was reinforced by the 2010 NIH Consensus Development Conference. Whether provision of access to VBAC should be considered an indicator of hospital maternal health care quality remains controversial. Although hospital VBAC rates were tracked as a quality measure until late 2007 by The Joint Commission as part of the Pregnancy and Related Conditions Care Measure Set, they are now considered to be neutral, meaning that internal hospital goals can be met by increases or decreases in VBAC rates.[36] Currently, The Joint Commission's Perinatal Care Core Measure Set includes cesarean rates, but no longer includes VBAC rates.[37]

Thus, largely before the 1999 ACOG recommendations, on both local and national levels, opinion leaders appeared able to promote the use of VBAC. As the numbers of women undergoing VBAC increased during the 1990's, and as studies clarifying the risks to VBAC were published and some opinion leaders voiced their concern, the VBAC rate began to decline. By 1999, with the ACOG Practice Bulletin publication,[27] the VBAC decline had become well established. ACOG is considered the ultimate opinion leader, and their professional guidelines largely describe the standard of care. Practicing physicians are held to that standard in the determination of liability in cases of medical malpractice. Thus, the connection between professional guidelines and practice patterns should be natural and strong. Although physicians can be heavily influenced by opinion leaders and guidelines, the data confirming the relationship between the VBAC decline and these events are sparse but compelling. Any impact of the 2010 conference on future VBAC rates remains unknown.

HOSPITAL FACILITIES AND IMMEDIATE CESAREAN AVAILABILITY

Given that hospitals no longer practicing VBAC seem to cite the 1999 ACOG guideline requiring immediate cesarean availability as a principal reason behind their decision to eliminate this practice, it is surprising that there has been little guidance from the literature establishing what is a safe environment for VBAC. From the reports by Shihady and colleagues[32] and Roberts and colleagues,[33] it seems that many hospital organizations do not believe they can meet the expected standard. If anesthesia personnel must be called in, operating rooms are being used, or blood bank services are limited, would these circumstances show the lack of immediate availability of emergency care? de Regt and colleagues[38] described the multiple factors in addition to physician availability, including operating room and anesthesia-related problems, affecting the time interval from cesarean decision to incision.

In addition to the few data providing evidence regarding what facilities make a hospital safe for VBAC, there is little evidence regarding operational policies that contribute to this safety. Nurse-staffing levels and physician availability in a VBAC environment have not been studied. What is the training required for both nurses and physicians to recognize the risks and complications of VBAC? Although the safety of the candidacy and medical management of VBAC itself has been extensively studied, and safety recommendations have been produced, following these recommendations to the letter may become moot in a hospital that is understaffed or lacks the resources to stabilize both mother and fetus within just a few minutes.

Individual hospitals must rely on their own assessment of what it would take, both in terms of facilities and policies, to meet the standard of immediate availability in emergency services. Some hospitals may find that they have always met such a standard, and need make no changes to their facilities or practices. Lavin and colleagues,[39] in a 2002 survey of Ohio hospitals performing VBAC, found that only 16% of level I hospitals had 24-hour availability of what they defined as complete emergency services: an obstetrician, in-house anesthesia, and a surgical team. These numbers increased to 63% in level II and 100% in level III hospitals. Level I and II hospitals increased staff when women desiring VBAC were present, but personnel were not routinely available.

There has been limited exploration of the types and ownership of hospitals that seem to have the highest VBAC rates,[3,23,40–47] and, although study designs for multi-hospital investigations differ greatly, it is generally conceded that university, tertiary care, and teaching hospitals with obstetric residency programs provide greatest access to TOLAC. Such hospitals are often staffed around the clock, and have full anesthesia and neonatal intensive care unit (NICU) services. Other types of hospitals, particularly rural and smaller community hospitals, may never be able to afford to achieve the immediate availability standard. Because delivery volume is so closely related to hospital ownership and level, its relationship to TOLAC access remains unclear.[47] Because VBAC success rates are fairly consistent across settings,[3,43,48] it is believed that hospital characteristics associated with VBAC largely reflect those hospitals providing access to TOLAC.

Although there have been some reports, little is known regarding how rural hospitals manage VBAC risk.[49–51] Community hospitals whose physicians are not employees or members of a contracted physician group may never be able to regulate or enforce physician availability. Although the latest available data indicate that most American women (99%) deliver in hospitals,[52] access to VBAC in birth centers remains hotly politicized[53,54] and, in one study, was shown to be associated with slightly higher risks compared with hospital birth.[55] Published studies regarding TOLAC with providers other than hospital-based obstetricians remain equivocal because of the lack of case-mix adjustment.[12]

There remains much unexplained variation in hospital TOLAC and VBAC rates, and further data collection and analysis at the hospital level, in addition to the patient level, are required to develop a more comprehensive understanding of hospital operations and the decision to provide access to a TOLAC. Studies of staffing structures, facility resources and capacity, business models, participation in hospital systems and networks, and malpractice insurance carrier restrictions should lead to an improved understanding of the hospital culture behind the VBAC decision. The wide variation in VBAC rates across (and within) the 50 states may, in large part, be caused by many of these issues, with more rural states, particularly in the South, having the lowest VBAC rates.[56]

This lack of evidence for what constitutes a safe VBAC environment is probably the most fundamental gap in the understanding of VBAC risks. What is a safe environment for VBAC both in terms of facilities and policies? How might this environment depend on hospital ownership and staffing structures? How should rural hospitals and birth centers coordinate care for women desiring VBAC? Now that medical risk has been fairly well defined, efforts should be directed at understanding and creating a safe and effective environment in which to conduct TOLAC. Potential considerations for perinatal policies for hospitals that allow VBAC are listed in **Box 1**.

REIMBURSEMENT FOR PROVIDING A TRIAL OF LABOR

Apart from concern regarding the facilities and policies needed to provide emergency services, there are also concerns about the resources spent on providing TOLAC. Historically, it has been assumed that ERCD would use more hospital resources

---

Box 1
Perinatal policies considered for hospitals that allow VBAC

1. Written informed consent

2. In-house anesthesia

3. Crash cesarean drills for all labor and delivery personnel and physicians practicing obstetrics

4. Requirement for all physicians who practice obstetrics to practice critical-events drills as a condition of reappointment to the medical staff

5. Ongoing education on the clinical signs and symptoms of uterine rupture

6. Ongoing education on the fetal monitoring signs of pending uterine rupture

7. Avoidance of induction of labor in patients having VBAC

---

than would a vaginal delivery. In 1997, Finkler and Wirtschafter[57] showed that variation in hospital cesarean rates appeared unrelated to variation in obstetric costs, and that obstetric costs depended more on staffing issues than mode of delivery. After 1989, Medicaid no longer paid a differential to physicians for cesarean delivery and, shortly thereafter, most insurance carriers followed suit.[58] Keeler and Fok[59] and Grant[58] have shown that this equalization of payment to physicians regardless of delivery method had little impact on the cesarean rate.

However, insurance payments to hospitals do seem to vary by delivery method, as indicated by the diagnosis-related groups (DRGs) associated with childbirth. DRGs, now reclassified as Medicare severity DRGs (MS-DRGs), are classifications for hospital admissions derived by the Medicare prospective payment system, indicating the amount Medicare pays to the hospital. For the fiscal year 2010 to 2011, the relative weights (RWs) for each of the childbirth-related DRGs are shown in **Table 2**.[60] The derivation of the RW for the DRG is largely based on total length of hospital stay. Thus, a higher length of stay generally yields a higher payment.

RWs are multiplied by a base rate (which is determined by regional labor costs and urban vs rural status). In fiscal year 2010, using simplified calculations, a typical base rate for an urban hospital would be $6732.[60] Given an RW of 0.50 for an uncomplicated vaginal delivery (eg, VBAC), the hospital payment would be approximately $3366; this compares with an RW of 0.75 for an uncomplicated cesarean delivery, yielding a hospital payment of $5049. Thus, such a difference in RW yields a hospital fee for the delivery of a woman with a prior cesarean by repeat cesarean that is 50% greater than that for a vaginal delivery. This increased hospital payment for

---

Table 2
MS-DRGs associated with childbirth and the relative weight assigned from the prospective payment system (version 27, fiscal year 2010)

MS-DRG	Relative Weight
765: cesarean with complications	1.11
766: cesarean without complications	0.75
774: vaginal delivery with complications	0.69
775: vaginal delivery without complications	0.50
767: vaginal delivery with sterilization	0.84
768: vaginal delivery with operating room procedure other than sterilization	1.78

cesarean delivery was confirmed in the statistical brief published by the Agency for Healthcare Research and Quality (AHRQ),[61] Hospitalizations Related to Childbirth, 2006, which used payer-derived data by DRG to calculate the mean cost of an uncomplicated vaginal delivery at $2600 compared with that of an uncomplicated cesarean delivery at $4500. Generally, the DRG rates are, directly or indirectly, the basis for hospital payment by the government and most medical insurance carriers. The degree to which hospitals accept DRG rates versus fixed payments for childbirth (perhaps derived from the DRG mix of the covered population), and how these payments might affect VBAC availability, remains unknown.

Clark and colleagues[62] published a convincing study showing that it was not likely to be profitable for a hospital to offer a TOLAC program. Only by using the most optimistic assumptions about the neonatal consequences after a uterine rupture, and a successful VBAC rate of 70%, could any savings be realized. In all other scenarios, from the perspective of a health care system, there was a net financial loss. Grobman and colleagues[63] also performed a cost-effectiveness study of ERCD versus TOLAC, using more detail and modeling immediate maternal morbidity and consequences to subsequent pregnancies. They concluded that a large number of cesareans with substantial maternal morbidity and expense would need to be performed to prevent 1 major adverse neonatal outcome (ie, number needed to treat). However, it seems that they grossly underestimated the cost of a child with cerebral palsy, and it is unclear to what degree this would have affected their results.[64,65] The contrast between these 2 studies illustrates the difficulty in estimating the cost of VBAC, and that the costs may accrue differently to different parties, whether they be third-party payers, parents, or society in general.

Nevertheless, if the focus is only on labor and delivery (where the decision regarding VBAC is ultimately made) women undergoing VBAC seem to require more immediate resources than do women undergoing elective repeat cesarean. In contrast with a woman with an unscarred uterus, a woman undergoing VBAC is expected to arrive at the hospital early in labor, and be placed on continuous fetal monitoring. She may therefore have a longer admission-to-delivery time, and require more nursing attention and vigilance. Zupancic,[66] in his review of the costs of elective cesarean delivery, notes cost differences ranging between $139[67] and $2294[68] between ERCD and TOLAC, but cautions that "comparison of elective cesarean section with a trial of labor may not yield cost savings, because a proportion of such trials lead to operative delivery, resulting in higher costs due to a longer duration of stay in labor and delivery, with its associated intensive personnel costs." He further notes that, in cost estimates of cesarean with and without labor, the latter were always higher.[66] Chung and colleagues[68] confirmed that "if the probability of successful vaginal birth after cesarean (VBAC) was less than 0.65, elective repeat cesarean was both less costly and more effective than a trial of labor." For women with a prior cesarean, Chung and colleagues[68] estimated the actual costs of a successful trial of labor ($3900–$6000), a failed trial of labor ($7000–$10,000), and ERCD ($5900–$8600). Obstetricians' services were given as $1450 to $1650 within these estimates. Given that physicians make roughly the same amount of money for vaginal and cesarean deliveries, convenience, time management, risk, and liability remain real, albeit as yet immeasurable, concerns. These studies collectively suggest that any immediate cost savings associated with a TOLAC program would be debatable.

Clark and colleagues[62] concluded that hospitals that provide VBAC are doing so with some motive other than saving money, and many hospitals providing VBAC do so with a community mission. However, insurers who pay DRG or global delivery rates seem to be getting a bargain with VBAC. To compound this bargain, insurers are also beginning to charge higher premiums to women with a prior cesarean, stating that the high probability of a repeat cesarean may cost them more.[69]

MEDICAL LIABILITY

Medical malpractice litigation and its costs have contributed sizably to the declining availability of VBAC.[70,71] According to the most recent ACOG liability survey,[72] nearly 91% of obstetrician-gynecologists reported involvement in at least 1 medical negligence claim in their career (average 2.7), 62% of the reported claims were for obstetrics, and 46% of these claims related to neurologic injury or death. Cohen and Schifrin[73] report that most obstetric lawsuits concern management of labor and delivery. Sixty percent of the ACOG survey respondents reported making changes to their practice because liability insurance is either unavailable or unaffordable. Of the 63% of the ACOG membership who reported making changes to their practice as a result of the risk or fear of liability claims or litigation, 30% decreased the number of high-risk obstetric patients that they accepted, 29% reported performing more cesareans, and 26% stopped offering/performing VBAC. Eight percent of survey respondents stopped practicing altogether. There has been much concern expressed about these trends and how they affect general access to childbirth services. Even a malpractice premium subsidy in Oregon does not seem to have stopped that state's continuing loss of maternity care providers.[74]

Obstetric malpractice premium rates, which have been negatively associated with VBAC rates, have continued to increase in recent years.[75] Premium rates vary tremendously by state because of state laws governing malpractice litigation.[76] For obstetricians, the average annual premium is about $50,000, although it may range from as low as $17,000 on average in states such as Oklahoma and Nebraska, to highs of $100,000 or more in states such as Florida and Nevada.[77]

From the physician perspective, VBAC is generally believed to be a safe procedure. Physicians and academicians are taught to examine risks in the aggregate, and, with the plethora of studies regarding VBAC risk, most would agree that the absolute risks are low and, as discussed earlier, must be viewed in the context of the risks of ERCD. As outlined in **Table 1**, the risks of repeat cesarean are largely to the mother, and are largely unpredictable. The risks of VBAC are largely to the fetus and are well known and quantifiable. Given the known 1% risk of uterine rupture, the ability to foresee harm and the consequent duty to prevent harm are legal concepts that are often used to prosecute a uterine rupture case.[78] However, a 1% risk of a uterine rupture does not necessarily make a uterine rupture foreseeable. Moreover, the ability to prevent harm from a VBAC depends primarily on whether the obstetrician and nurses who are conducting the VBAC are on notice of a uterine rupture in progress. As described earlier, notice relates to the circumstances in which the physician and nurses have sufficient time to identify the potential for a uterine rupture and ample opportunity to deliver the patient.[31] In the case of a uterine rupture, the greater duty for the physician and/or nurse to prevent fetal injury arises when the providers are on notice of the uterine rupture by virtue of the changes in the fetal heart rate pattern and/or maternal signs and symptoms. In the absence of notice, and where there is no warning that a uterine rupture is about to occur, the physician and the nurse are less able to prevent the death or disability of the fetus.

Medical malpractice litigation in VBAC cases has also incorporated the concept that a procedure, such as VBAC, or a device, may be considered inherently dangerous. Inherently dangerous typically means a condition of ever-present hazard requiring special precautions to avoid damage or injury. The concept of inherent danger arises from product liability actions and relates to the hazardous properties of a manufactured device. Here, the practice of VBAC may be likened to an inherently dangerous product or procedure. In the case of brain-damaged baby from a uterine rupture, the concept of inherently dangerous can be argued because the risk of uterine rupture is estimated to be 18 times higher in a prior cesarean patient and the window to prevent injury is said to be 18 minutes, or less in some circumstances. To date, the obstetric profession has argued that VBAC is not inherently dangerous in the presence of immediately available cesarean services; however, studies have not tested whether such a standard will prevent all harm.

Assumption of the risk is another legal concept that applies primarily to the patient and her willingness to accept certain procedures such as a VBAC, operative vaginal delivery, or a cesarean. The typical way to transfer the risk of medical procedures, and have the patient assume the risk, is through informed consent.[79] Informed consent is considered whenever medical alternatives exist. A patient with a prior cesarean has alternatives with respect to route of delivery. In general, this means that the obstetrician has an obligation to explain the options and downstream consequences of each option to the patient and let her make a choice. By so doing, she assumes the risks of the option selected. With proper informed consent, the patient assumes the risk of nonnegligent care. The patient cannot assume the risk of negligent care, nor can she necessarily assume the risks for the fetus. In all cases, it remains the prerogative of the providers of care to determine whether they can provide VBAC safely, and both doctors and hospitals may decline to provide VBAC services.

Further contextualizing the concept of VBAC risk are the legal consequences of VBAC-related morbidity. Although the absolute risks to VBAC may be small, the financial consequences of a maloccurrence can be enormous, with evidence that the median award for medical negligence in childbirth cases is now $2.3 million.[80] Clark and colleagues[81] presented an analysis of 189 closed claims between 2000 and 2005, of which 10 (5.3%) were VBAC related, with an average payment of about $1 million per case. In the ACOG liability survey, more than half the obstetric cases reported seemed to have been settled without any payment on behalf of the obstetrician but, regardless of financial payout, the personal costs to the individual providers in terms of time and anxiety can be devastating. Because a VBAC may be considered inherently risky, these results indicate that many cases may be without merit, often with parents seeking compensation because they need financial assistance to care for a brain-injured child. An estimate made by the Centers for Disease Control in 1992, found the cost of a child with cerebral palsy to be about a half-million dollars.[64] The development of state-wide risk pools to compensate parents for their child's needs and avoid a malpractice suit has shown some usefulness.[82,83] Brennan and colleagues[84] reported that the severity of the patient's disability, not the occurrence of an adverse event or an adverse event caused by negligence, was predictive of payment to the plaintiff. Given that the worst outcomes of uterine rupture are fetal brain injury and death, and that these can occur even in circumstances that would not be considered negligent, it is understandable why, despite the rarity of uterine rupture, VBAC liability is so high and VBAC rates continue to be low.

PATIENT-LEVEL FACTORS

In the last few years, the concept of the ideal VBAC candidate has narrowed to that of a woman with 1 prior cesarean with a low, transverse uterine scar.[1] The extent to which a smaller candidate pool may be contributing to a lower number of women choosing a TOLAC is unknown. Factors contributing to the likelihood of success are a prior vaginal birth and presentation in spontaneous labor.[10] Factors mitigating against success are a recurrent indication for initial cesarean, increased maternal age, nonwhite ethnicity, gestational age greater than 40 weeks, maternal obesity, preeclampsia, short interpregnancy interval, and increased neonatal birth weight[10]; many of these conditions are becoming increasingly prevalent.[85] Women receive counseling from their providers, and the extent to which the informed consent process reflects provider preferences, biases, or health system limitations is unknown. What is clear, given falling VBAC attempt rates, is that an increasing number of women seem discouraged from attempting VBAC.

Whether insurance issues or racial disparities are influencing TOLAC rates remains uncertain because of strong correlations among race, insurance, and hospital ownership. Most studies have not examined these relationships using hierarchical models that can account for these interactions. Using hierarchical models that separate out effects at the patient and hospital levels, the authors have found no relationship of TOLAC to insurance type,[4,45,86] although it does seem (as discussed earlier) to be related to hospital type, with Health Maintenance Organization and tertiary hospitals most likely to offer a TOLAC. VBAC success does not seem to be related to patient insurance type, although there have been several conflicting studies with different methodologies and different correlated variables.[12,87,88] Nonwhite race seems negatively related to VBAC success, but not to TOLAC[89,90]; nonwhite race has been postulated to have a negative clinical impact but not to be a factor that decreases access to VBAC. However, the length of TOLAC, and the clinical management of patients, may vary with both racial or insurance characteristics, but there is no evidence that supports such conjecture. Kramer and colleagues[12] suggest that: "In theory, differences observed could occur for one of several reasons, including differential provision of information to subpopulations; increased acceptance of recommendations by providers by subpopulations; cultural differences in the importance of vaginal delivery; and differences in the level of provider experience with subpopulations."

In the report of its national survey in 2006, Listening to Mothers, Childbirth Connection documented that 11% of women with a prior cesarean had a vaginal delivery with their most recent birth, although 45% of them had been interested in a VBAC.[91] Of these women, 57% stated that they were denied that option. When asked what reason was given for the denial of a VBAC, the leading responses were unwillingness of their caregiver (45%) or the hospital (23%), followed by a medical reason unrelated to the prior cesarean (20%). In addition, anecdotal stories exist of women with histories of prior cesarean delivery arriving at hospitals in a state of imminent delivery being taken for immediate repeat cesarean, not having had the benefit of informed consent or being given the option to push. Melnikow and colleagues[92] corroborated these findings in a California study showing that many hospital records for patients with a prior cesarean lacked evidence of counseling regarding a TOLAC. These reports are in keeping with the physician's and hospital's right not to participate in a VBAC. However, the article by Melnikow and colleagues[92] is disquieting because the importance of VBAC informed consent had been recognized for more than a decade.[22] The absence of documented informed consent raises the question regarding the extent to which women are choosing ERCD, and to what extent the system is choosing this option for them; how much autonomy do women have regarding the VBAC decision?

The apparent erosion of patient autonomy in obstetrics has raised many concerns.[80,93–95] The ACOG Practice Bulletin acknowledges that patient preferences should be considered, particularly when the risks associated with the choice of ERCD and TOLAC seem equivalent.[9] It is also widely speculated that patient preferences may be contributing to the decline in VBAC attempts, because there is some evidence that patients are becoming more risk averse, and are becoming more comfortable with the repeat cesarean choice.[96,97] This trend has been attributed to the generally acknowledged maternal perspective of placing greater value on the risk to the fetus than the risk to herself.[98] Given the recent acceptance of maternal-request cesarean delivery within the obstetric community,[99,100] it is not surprising that many patients should see ERCD as a preferable option. However, the health consequences and practice implications of allowing maternal preference alone to dictate the use of cesarean are not fully understood.[94]

Some investigators have attempted to describe the issues associated with the integration of patient preferences into the VBAC decision. It may seem that patients and physicians end up talking past each other when it comes to the risk equation. Aspects of birth valued by patients are not necessarily taken into account when the risks are explained.[98,101] For example, a patient may prefer to have a VBAC because the lesser morbidity would enable her to better care for her children.[102] Family and work issues may play a prominent role in a woman's decisions, but are not routinely included in risk discussions. The degree to which patients' current and future concerns affect their decision shows that women use a wider context than the absolute risk when assessing the risk of VBAC. How to educate women and help them arrive at a decision is currently being studied, but there is little clear guidance at present.[103–107]

The VBAC decision shows the conflict common to many patients who try to navigate the health care system. As our insurance and health delivery systems become more complex, as medical care becomes more specialized, and as the evaluation of both system and provider performance becomes a science in itself, consumers require more knowledge and greater skill to take full advantage of new sources of information and to make informed choices.[108] Health literacy, or the ability to make these informed choices, has been recognized as a national imperative through both the Institute of Medicine and AHRQ reports in 2004.[109,110] These choices are especially relevant to women making a VBAC decision because of the difficulty, as outlined in this article, in understanding both the medical risk and the hospital environment.

In these circumstances, women must often use doctors as agents to help them with such choices because there are few other avenues to understand which services are safest and which suit them best.[111] This concept of agency has long substituted for a lack of public accounting by our health care services.[112] Patients place trust in their physicians to guide them, but physician agency is itself imperfect because it is subject to business interests and efficiencies.[113] To most consumers, public data regarding the cost and quality of health care services can seem unintelligible and irrelevant.[114] The development of performance metrics, although highly touted, remains rudimentary, as the subtleties, dynamics, and controversies of what truly is quality health care become more and more apparent.[115]

An example of this dilemma is that women who enter the hospital with birth plans (specified, legitimate options regarding use of epidurals, ambulation, intravenous lines, episiotomies, cesareans), tend to have the same interventions as other women without explicit choices delivering in the same hospital.[95,116] Medical circumstances may require unexpected interventions during childbirth, but the culture and efficiencies within hospital practices tend to remain dominant.

This phenomenon is well identified in the consumer-choice literature as the gap between what consumers say they want and the services they receive.[117,118] Consumers may have awareness and comprehension of quality and safety differences, they may even have beliefs and attitudes that support making appropriate choices, but they often do not use services wisely. Whether the reason for uninformed choice is at the consumer level (eg, with respect to motivation, need for proximity or services, or perceived cost of alternatives) or whether it is at the agency or service level (eg, physician, hospital, or insurer) remains to be explored.

The question remains, are women themselves less convinced that VBAC is a reasonable option, or are they being dissuaded by the health care system? Most women giving birth do have a choice of caregivers and facilities, although exceptions are those who have a pregnancy complication and need specialized care,[119] those who live in isolated or rural areas,[120] and those who have insurance limitations. Choices for women with public insurance appeared to increase greatly in the early 1990s as mechanisms for hospital reimbursement allowed public patients to be cared for at private hospitals.[121]

Are women desiring VBAC unwilling, or unable, to choose childbirth providers and hospitals that believe they can safely provide this service? Are they willing to go farther from home to get a TOLAC? In general, hospital choices are largely determined by convenience of location, which may or may not be directly related to proximity.[122,123] Local hospitals tend to be used in emergencies and by the elderly and the indigent, in particular.[121] However, many patients, including pregnant women,[124] commonly go outside their local areas for hospital services. They seem to be most influenced by the perceived quality of these services and the need for more specialized services.[120,122,125,126]

Patients appreciate having choices with respect to their hospitals, and, although greater choice does not always lead to greater satisfaction with health care services,[127–129] this choice contributes to the subjective experience of empowerment,[130] which is intrinsic to the mechanism of health care decision making. Furthermore, patients seem willing to make trade-offs with respect to hospitals more easily than with other health care decisions, perhaps because hospitals can be more easily viewed as accountable for their services, in contrast with health plans or provider networks.[131]

Although hospitals vary widely in their outcomes for both mothers and newborns, most women are not aware that such wide differences in services exist.[91] For example, in California, among laboring nulliparous women with normal pregnancies, 29% of mother-newborn pairs suffered at least 1 serious childbirth complication such as infection or birth trauma.[132] This rate varied from 9% to 76% among hospitals, and did not include cesarean delivery, which itself varied between 4% and 40% in this low-risk population at the hospitals studied.[132] Facilities, services, resources, and policies also vary widely across childbirth hospitals, but there is no systematic way for women to determine the optimal environment for their labor and delivery. The NIH Consensus Conference Statement on VBAC recognized this important point, and recommended that "health care organizations, physicians, and other clinicians should consider making public their trial of labor policies and VBAC rates, as well as their plans for responding to obstetric emergencies."[1]

In summary, the increasing prevalence and recognition of clinical characteristics that may put women and their fetuses at increased risk from VBAC are likely to be contributing to decreased candidacy for TOLAC, and, thus, lower VBAC rates. However, it remains unclear how the VBAC decision is being made, and the degree to which the declining use of VBAC reflects women's preferences, their use of their physicians as agents to make this decision, or the lack of nearby facilities to safely undergo VBAC. A better understanding is needed of how to incorporate patient preferences into childbirth services, and increased transparency on the part of the health care system. Furthermore, there is increasing recognition that patients need more than the mere transmission of information and that they require the development of skills and confidence to make choices.[133]

CONSIDERATIONS FOR A RESEARCH AGENDA

The NIH Consensus Conference noted several critical gaps in the evidence required for decision making about VBAC, and included limited understanding of a variety of nonmedical factors affecting the availability and management of TOLAC.[1] They specifically observed that access to a safe trial of labor seems to be restricted by factors such as geography, workforce availability and training, professional association guidelines, type of maternity care provider, liability concerns, health insurance, and institutional policy. They recommended well-designed studies to better understand these factors and to test clinical, institutional, or policy interventions to increase access to a safe trial of labor. They also noted the necessity for the development of interventions to reduce the barrier of professional liability, and the further development of decision-making tools to assist in the informed consent process.

In addition to these recommendations, this review would emphasize that a fundamental concept is lacking within the VBAC evidence base: there is little understanding of the components of a safe environment for VBAC. The facilities, staffing, and operational and policy structures that support optimal outcomes for both the mother and fetus have received little attention in the VBAC debate. The focus has been on clinical risk, which, although important, comprises only an chapter (albeit a very relevant chapter) in the story of the VBAC decline. ACOG has carefully defined safe practices around TOLAC, but there is little guidance, and even less evidence, regarding what constitutes a safe environment.

To further the obstetric community's understanding of what makes a safe environment for VBAC will naturally require the study and comparison of a variety of childbirth environments. In contrast with other clinical areas such as cardiology, in which mandatory reporting of outcomes has led to the evolution of detailed data collection systems that have allowed extensive exploration of quality and safety issues, obstetric data systems both within and across hospital systems remain rudimentary and lack standardization. At more than 4 million births per year in the United States, childbirth is the number 1 reason for hospital admission,[134] and this vast pool of data is largely relegated to paper charts. Those hospital systems with electronic medical records (EMRs), although often a step ahead of those without, require complex technical efforts and often a nonexistent budget to standardize data, create reports, and track outcomes. Although data elements such as a history of a prior cesarean may be easily found in the EMR, these records do not usually lend themselves to identifying fundamental patient characteristics such as the presence of labor, or pregnancy and obstetric complications.

In addition to the obstetric community's reliance on administrative data (ie, International Classification of Diseases, Version 9, Clinical Modification [ICD-9-CM] codes), the use of EMR data could offer more process information (ie, practice information about the actual conduct of labor and delivery) and would assist in the examination and determination of best practices. One example is cesarean decision-incision time. Cardiologists have examined and tried to improve door-to-balloon time for many years.[135] Although independent efforts have been made to improve decision-incision times in obstetrics,[38,136] there is little standardized documentation in obstetrics for such process measures, and this situation is unlikely to change unless backed by a strong commitment within the obstetric and quality improvement communities.

Given the low risks of many of the pertinent outcomes of TOLAC, extensive data collection is required to gain sufficient statistical power to address the safety issues across multihospital settings. The obstetric community may need to explore the greater use of registries and conduct more studies in regional hospital systems that have consistent, standardized, and validated data collection mechanisms. Furthermore, more complex statistical methods, such as hierarchical modeling, are required to accurately assess the significance of patient and hospital factors and separately account for within-hospital and between-hospital variability in outcomes. There remains little understanding of how a trial of labor may proceed for different patient subgroups (eg, based on insurance and race/ethnicity), and how this may vary by hospital setting.

A second fundamental task, as evidence is developed regarding what is a safe VBAC environment, is to determine how to develop operational systems to create and implement such an environment. Such efforts will rely heavily on regional collaborative strategies for sharing information and services. This reliance means that the obstetric community must work with all stakeholders (ie, physicians, hospitals, patients, attorneys, policy makers, payers, and employers) to develop realistic strategies that address both clinical and nonclinical concerns. How do women identify and access this safe environment? Can delivery payment be uncoupled from prenatal care so that physicians are willing to transfer mothers for delivery, if necessary? What incentives are there for physicians to transfer patients? Can there be more equity or incentives in payment for hospitals to provide TOLAC? What type of staff education, policies, and leadership are needed at the hospital level to make the organizational advances needed to put safety first? What can rural hospitals do to enhance TOLAC safety?

Although the goal of medical liability reform seems unreachable, some have suggested the implementation of binding arbitration to adjudicate negligence claims derived from adverse outcomes of high-risk obstetric procedures, suggesting that "patient autonomy is violated far more profoundly by forcing VBAC-eligible women to deliver through cesarean than by implementing binding arbitration using a public, fair and transparent arbitration board as a mechanism to save VBAC from extinction."[80]

If the obstetric community is serious about providing a safe environment for the wide-ranging risks encountered in obstetrics in general, and in particular for the VBAC decision, it may require the thorough investigation of the specific facilities, staffing, and policies pertinent to each obstetric risk category. For example, regionalized NICU systems specifically outline where mothers should deliver so that the appropriate services are available depending on medical needs and gestational age. Enough evidence has accumulated to show that regionalization of these services does provide neonatal benefit and improved safety.[137-140]

There has not been similar progress in defining levels of obstetric care that would provide safety to mothers.[141] It seems that the obstetric community has settled on cesarean delivery as the common denominator so that routine hospital practices are not restricted. Thus, many established obstetric interventions are now steadily disappearing: operative vaginal delivery, particularly forceps; external cephalic version, vaginal delivery of twin gestations, especially with malpresentation of twin B; and a trial of labor for marginal placenta previa.[80,94] This default position, to allow all hospitals to provide all services for all mothers with reliance on neonatal transport as necessary on delivery, has its own consequences, and likely has contributed to the overwhelming increase in cesarean delivery and the elimination of other, potentially riskier, delivery options. If a wider variety of obstetric practices is to be preserved, then consideration should be given to the creation and credentialing of those environments that can safely manage the additional risk. At this time, some hospital administrators are concluding that they cannot provide a safe environment for VBAC, and opt instead for ERCD. Instead of arriving at this conclusion by default, it would be helpful to have the data to support and guide the creation of standards for risk levels of obstetric care.

The third fundamental task of the research agenda would be to encourage hospitals to strengthen their obstetric information systems and to begin to provide the transparency that is so essential for women and other stakeholders to begin to develop the skills and the context for making decisions regarding VBAC. Process and outcomes transparency requires proactive leadership within organizations that have historically functioned as a collection of silos, with largely independent and overworked staff, and immature organizational infrastructure.[142,143] Such transparency contains a high degree of risk to the stability of the health care organization itself; for example, the risk that suboptimal practices will be discovered by others, risk of medical liability, and risk that corrective workflow changes (and their associated expenses) will be mandated for a system that is already strained.[144]

Women's dependence on physician agency to determine delivery choices might be lessened if hospitals were able to provide and share information about policies, facilities, practices, and outcomes. What is a hospital's average decision-incision time for emergency cesareans? What kind of training does a hospital staff undergo to manage TOLAC? Can feasible and interpretable indicators of hospital childbirth quality care be developed? If there is such wide variation across hospitals regarding complication rates for normal births, trying to give women meaningful information about differences in the risks of TOLAC will involve an even greater effort.

SUMMARY

The use of TOLAC has persistently declined in the last decade, although medical risks to TOLAC, although now better defined, remain low and essentially unchanged. Factors contributing to the nonclinical context of TOLAC are pervasive and strong, and must be considered in any strategy to increase TOLAC rates. Principal among these factors are ACOG's recommendation for immediately available cesarean services, which is cited as a major reason why hospitals no longer provide VBAC. The development of an evidence base to provide guidance regarding the policies, staffing, and facilities needed to create a safe environment for VBAC, and organizational strategies for implementing the components of this environment, should be vigorously pursued. The development of obstetric information systems that can provide safety and quality information is critical to this effort.

REFERENCES

1. National Institutes of Health. National Institutes of Health Consensus Development Conference statement: vaginal birth after cesarean: new insights, March 8-10, 2010. Obstet Gynecol 2010;115(6):1279–95.
2. Martin JA, Hamilton BE, Sutton PD, et al. Births: final data for 2007. Natl Vital Stat Rep 2010;58(24):1–125.
3. Gregory KD, Fridman M, Korst L. Trends and patterns of vaginal birth after cesarean availability in the United States. Semin Perinatol 2010;34:237–43.
4. Gregory KD, Korst LM, Gornbein JA, et al. Using administrative data to identify indications for elective cesarean delivery. Health Serv Res 2002;37:1387–401.
5. DeFrances CJ, Cullen KA, Kozak LJ. National Center for Health Statistics. National Hospital Discharge Survey. 2005 annual summary with detailed diagnosis and procedure data. Vital Health Stat 13 2007;(165):1–209.
6. National Institutes of Health. Cesarean childbirth. National Institutes of Health consensus statement online 1980;3(6):1–30. Available at: http://consensus.nih.gov/1980/1980Cesarean027html.htm. Accessed December 1, 2010.

7. Cohen B, Atkins M. Brief history of vaginal birth after cesarean section. Clin Obstet Gynecol 2001;44:604–8.
8. Riva HL, Teich JC. Vaginal delivery after cesarean section. Am J Obstet Gynecol 1961;81:501–10.
9. Landon MB. Vaginal birth after cesarean delivery. Clin Perinatol 2008;35: 491–504.
10. American College of Obstetricians and Gynecologists (ACOG). Vaginal birth after previous cesarean delivery. ACOG Practice Bulletin number 115, August 2010. Obstet Gynecol 2010;116(2 Part 1):450–63.
11. Guise JM, Denman MA, Emeis C, et al. Vaginal birth after cesarean: new insights on maternal and neonatal outcomes. Obstet Gynecol 2010;115(6):1267–78.
12. Kraemer DF, Berlin M, Guise JM. The relationship of health care delivery system characteristics and legal factors to mode of delivery in women with prior cesarean section: a systematic review. Womens Health Issues 2004;14:94–103.
13. Guise J-M, Eden K, Emeis C, et al. Vaginal birth after cesarean: new insights. evidence report/technology assessment No.191. AHRQ Publication No. 10-E003. Rockville (MD): Agency for Healthcare Research and Quality; 2010.
14. Lomas J, Enkin M, Anderson GM, et al. Opinion leaders vs audit and feedback to implement practice guidelines. Delivery after previous cesarean section. JAMA 1991;265(17):2202–7.
15. Lomas J, Anderson GM, Domnick-Pierre K, et al. Do practice guidelines guide practice? The effect of a consensus statement on the practice of physicians. N Engl J Med 1989;321(19):1306–11.
16. Santerre RE. The effect of the ACOG guideline on vaginal births after cesarean. Med Care Res Rev 1996;53(3):315–29.
17. Misra A. Impact of the HealthChoice program on cesarean section and vaginal birth after C-section deliveries: a retrospective analysis. Matern Child Health J 2008;12(2):266–74.
18. Yap OW, Kim ES, Laros RK Jr. Maternal and neonatal outcomes after uterine rupture in labor. Am J Obstet Gynecol 2001;184:1576–81.
19. Smith GC, Pell JP, Pasupathy D, et al. Factors predisposing to perinatal death related to uterine rupture during attempted vaginal birth after caesarean section: retrospective cohort study. BMJ 2004;329:375.
20. Zinberg S. Vaginal delivery after previous cesarean delivery: a continuing controversy. Clin Obstet Gynecol 2001;44(3):561–70.
21. American College of Obstetricians and Gynecologists (ACOG). ACOG Committee Statement. Guidelines for vaginal delivery after a cesarean childbirth. Washington, DC: ACOG; 1982.
22. Phelan JP. VBAC: time to reconsider? OBG Manage 1996;8(11):62, 64-8.
23. McMahon MJ, Luther ER, Bowes WA, et al. Comparison of a trial of labor with an elective second cesarean section. N Engl J Med 1996;335:689–95.
24. Flamm B. Point/counterpoint I. VBAC the pros. Obstet Gynecol Surv 1998; 53(11):658–61.
25. Phelan JP. Point/counterpoint: II. The VBAC "Con" Game. Obstet Gynecol Surv 1998;53(11):661–3.
26. Leung AS, Leung EK, Paul RH. Uterine rupture after previous cesarean delivery: maternal and fetal consequences. Am J Obstet Gynecol 1993;169: 945–50.
27. American College of Obstetricians and Gynecologists (ACOG). Vaginal birth after cesarean delivery. ACOG Practice Bulletin, No. 5, July 1999. Int J Gynaecol Obstet 1999;66:197–204.

28. Bayer-Zwirello LA, O'Grady JP, Patel SS. ACOG's 1999 VBAC Guidelines: a survey of western Massachusetts obstetric services. Obstet Gynecol 2000; 95(Suppl 4):73S.

29. Guidelines for perinatal care. 6th edition. Elk Grove Village (IL): American Academy of Pediatrics; 2007. p. 159.

30. American College of Obstetricians and Gynecologists (ACOG). Vaginal birth after previous cesarean delivery. ACOG Practice Bulletin No. 54. Obstet Gynecol 2004;104:203–12.

31. Phelan JP. Perinatal risk management: obstetric methods to prevent birth asphyxia. Clin Perinatol 2005;32:1–17.

32. Shihady IR, Broussard P, Bolton LB, et al. Vaginal birth after cesarean: do California hospital policies follow national guidelines? J Reprod Med 2007;52: 349–58.

33. Roberts RG, Deutchman M, King VJ, et al. Changing policies on vaginal birth after cesarean: impact on access. Birth 2007;34(4):316–22.

34. Gochnour G, Ratcliffe S, Stone MB. The Utah VBAC Study. Matern Child Health J 2005;9:1–8.

35. California Hospital Assessment and Reporting Taskforce. Available at: https://chart.ucsf.edu/. Accessed December 1, 2010.

36. The Joint Commission. General public quality report user guide: a guide to using the joint commission hospital accreditation quality report, 2008. Available at: http://www.qualitycheck.org/help_user_guides.aspx. Accessed December 1, 2010.

37. The Joint Commission. Perinatal care core measure set. Available at: https://manual.jointcommission.org/bin/view/Manual/WebHome. Accessed December 1, 2010.

38. de Regt RH, Marks K, Joseph DL, et al. Time from decision to incision for cesarean deliveries at a community hospital. Obstet Gynecol 2009;113:625–9.

39. Lavin JP, DePasquale L, Crane S, et al. A state-wide assessment of the obstetric, anesthesia, and operative team personnel who are available to manage the labors and deliveries and to treat the complications of women who attempt vaginal birth after cesarean delivery. Am J Obstet Gynecol 2002; 187:611–4.

40. Stafford RS. The impact of nonclinical factors on repeat cesarean section. JAMA 1991;265(1):59–63.

41. Gregory KD, Ramicone E, Chan L, et al. Cesarean deliveries for Medicaid patients: a comparison in public and private hospitals in Los Angeles County. Am J Obstet Gynecol 1990;180(5):1177–84.

42. Shiono PH, Fielden JG, McNellis D, et al. Recent trends in cesarean birth and trial of labor rates in the United States. JAMA 1987;257(4):494–7.

43. DeFranco EA, Rampersad R, Atkins KL, et al. Do vaginal birth after cesarean outcomes differ based on hospital setting? Am J Obstet Gynecol 2007;197: 400.e1–6.

44. Dunsmoor-Su R, Sammel M, Stevens E, et al. Impact of sociodemographic and hospital factors on attempts at vaginal birth after cesarean delivery. Obstet Gynecol 2003;102:1358–65.

45. Gregory KD, Korst LM, Cane P, et al. Vaginal birth after cesarean and uterine rupture rates in California. Obstet Gynecol 1999;94:985–9.

46. King DE, Lahiri K. Socioeconomic factors and the odds of vaginal birth after cesarean delivery. JAMA 1994;272(7):524–9.

47. Chang JJ, Stamilio DM, Macones GA. Effect of hospital volume on maternal outcomes in women with prior cesarean delivery undergoing trial of labor. Am J Epidemiol 2008;167:711–8.

48. Yeh J, Wactawski-Wende J, Shelton J, et al. Temporal trends in the rates of trial of labor in low risk pregnancies and their impact on the rates and success of vaginal birth after cesarean delivery. Am J Obstet Gynecol 2006;194(1): 144.e1–12.

49. Walton DL, Ludlow D, Willis DC. Vaginal birth after cesarean section: acceptance and outcome at a rural hospital. J Reprod Med 1993;38(9):716–8.

50. Raynor BD. The experience with vaginal birth after cesarean delivery in a small rural community practice. Am J Obstet Gynecol 1993;168(1 Pt 1):60–2.

51. Pinette MG, Kahn J, Gross KL, et al. Vaginal birth after cesarean rates are declining rapidly in the rural state of Maine. J Matern Fetal Neonatal Med 2004;16(1):37–43.

52. MacDorman MF, Menacker F, Declercq E. Trends and characteristics of home and other out-of-hospital births in the United States, 1990-2006. Natl Vital Stat Rep 2010;58(11):1–15.

53. Stratton B. 50 ways to protest a VBAC denial. Midwifery Today Int Midwife 2006; 78:28–9, 68-9.

54. Clark A. RH Reality Check. Challenge to Florida VBAC ban intensifies. Available at: http://www.rhrealitycheck.org/node/13213. Accessed December 1, 2010.

55. Lieberman E, Ernst EK, Rooks JP, et al. Results of the national study of vaginal birth after cesarean in birth centers. Obstet Gynecol 2004;104(5 Part 1):933–42.

56. Clarke SC, Taffel SM. State variation in rates of cesarean and VBAC delivery: 1989 and 1993. Stat Bull Metrop Insur Co 1996;77(1):28–36.

57. Finkler MD, Wirtschafter DD. One health maintenance organization's experience: obstetric costs depend more on staffing than on mode of delivery. J Perinatol 1997;17(2):148–55.

58. Grant D. Physician financial incentives and cesarean delivery: new conclusions from the healthcare cost and utilization project. J Health Econ 2009;28(1): 244–50.

59. Keeler E, Fok T. Equalizing physician fees had little effect on cesarean rates. Med Care Res Rev 1996;53(4):465–71.

60. Centers for Medicare and Medicaid Services (CMS) fiscal year 2010 final rule home page. Available at: http://www.cms.gov/AcuteInpatientPPS/10FR/itemdetail.asp? filterType=none&filterByDID=99&sortByDID=1&sortOrder=ascending&itemID= CMS1227477&intNumPerPage=10. Accessed December 1, 2010.

61. Russo CA, Weir L, Steiner C. Hospitalizations related to childbirth, 2006. HCUP statistical brief #71. Rockville (MD): US Agency for Healthcare Research and Quality; 2009. Available at: http://www.hcupus.ahrq.gov/reports/statbriefs/sb71. pdf. Accessed December 1, 2010.

62. Clark SL, Scott JR, Porter TF, et al. Is vaginal birth after cesarean less expensive than repeat cesarean delivery? Am J Obstet Gynecol 2000;182:599–602.

63. Grobman WA, Peaceman AM, Socol ML. Cost-effectiveness of elective cesarean delivery after one prior low transverse cesarean. Obstet Gynecol 2000;95:745–51.

64. Centers for Disease Control. Economic costs of birth defects and cerebral palsy–United States, 1992. MMWR Morb Mortal Wkly Rep 1995;44:694–9.

65. November MT. Cost analysis of vaginal birth after cesarean. Clin Obstet Gynecol 2001;44(3):571–87.

66. Zupancic JA. The economics of elective cesarean delivery. Clin Perinatol 2008; 35(3):591–9.

67. Bost BW. Cesarean delivery on demand: what will it cost? Am J Obstet Gynecol 2003;188:1418–21.

68. Chung A, Macario A, El-Sayed YY, et al. Cost-effectiveness of a trial of labor after previous cesarean. Obstet Gynecol 2001;97:932–41.
69. Grady D. Trying to avoid 2nd cesarean: many women find choice isn't theirs. NY Times November 29, 2004. p. A1. Available at: http://www.nytimes.com/2008/06/01/health/01insure.html. Accessed December 1, 2010.
70. Localio AR, Lawthers AG, Bengston JM, et al. Relationship between malpractice claims and cesarean delivery. JAMA 1993;269(3):366–73.
71. Murthy K, Grobman WA, Lee TA, et al. Association between rising professional liability insurance premiums and primary cesarean delivery rates. Obstet Gynecol 2007;110(6):1264–9.
72. American Congress of Obstetricians and Gynecologists (ACOG). ACOG releases 2009 medical liability survey. results paint dismal reality for ob-gyns and their patients. Available at: http://www.acog.org/from_home/publications/press_releases/nr09-11-09.cfm. Accessed December 1, 2010.
73. Cohen WR, Schifrin BS. Medical negligence lawsuits relating to labor and delivery. Clin Perinatol 2007;34:345–60.
74. Smits AK, King VJ, Rdesinski RE, et al. Change in Oregon maternity care workforce after malpractice premium subsidy implementation. Health Serv Res 2009;44(4):1253–70.
75. Yang YT, Mello MM, Subramanian SV, et al. Relationship between malpractice litigation pressure and rates of cesarean section and vaginal birth after cesarean. Med Care 2009;47(2):234–42.
76. Norton SA. The malpractice premium costs of obstetrics. Inquiry 1997;34(1):62–9.
77. Robinson P, Xu X, Keeton K, et al. The impact of medical legal risk on obstetrician-gynecologist supply. Obstet Gynecol 2005;105:1296–302.
78. Phelan JP, Korst LM, Martin GI. Causation – fetal brain injury and uterine rupture. Clin Perinatol 2007;34:409–38.
79. Phelan JP. Informed consent and medicolegal problems. Global Library of Womens Medicine (ISSN: 1756-2228). 2008. Available at: http://www.glowm.com/index.html?p=glowm.cml/section_view&articleid=73&recordset=Search%20results&value=. Accessed December 1, 2010.
80. Rybak EA. Hippocratic ideal, Faustian bargain and Damocles' sword: erosion of patient autonomy in obstetrics. J Perinatol 2009;29:721–5.
81. Clark SL, Belfort MA, Dildy GA, et al. Reducing obstetric litigation through alterations in practice patterns. Obstet Gynecol 2008;112(6):1279–83.
82. Stalnaker BL, Maher JE, Kleinman GE, et al. Characteristics of successful claims for payment by the Florida neurologic injury compensation association fund. Am J Obstet Gynecol 1997;177:268–73.
83. Florida Birth-Related Neurological Injury Compensation Association. Available at: http://www.nica.com/. Accessed December 1, 2010.
84. Brennan TA, Sox CM, Burstin HR. Relation between negligent adverse events and the outcomes of medical-malpractice litigation. N Engl J Med 1996;335:1963–7.
85. Srinivas SK, Epstein AJ, Nicholson S, et al. Improvements in US maternal obstetrical outcomes from 1992 to 2006. Med Care 2010;48(5):487–93.
86. Korst LM, Gornbein JA, Gregory KD. Rethinking the cesarean rate: how pregnancy complications may affect inter-hospital comparisons. Med Care 2005;43(3):237–45.
87. Oleske DM, Linn ES, Nachman KL, et al. Cesarean and VBAC delivery rates in Medicaid managed care, Medicaid fee for service, and private managed care. Birth 1998;25:125–7.

88. Wagner CL, Metts AK. Rates of successful vaginal delivery after cesarean for patients with private versus public insurance. J Perinatol 1999;1:14–8.

89. Hollard AL, Wing DA, Chung JH, et al. Ethnic disparity in the success of vaginal birth after cesarean. J Matern Fetal Neonat Med 2006;19(8):483–7.

90. Cahill AG, Stamilio DM, Odibo AO, et al. Racial disparity in the success and complications of vaginal birth after cesarean delivery. Obstet Gynecol 2008; 111(3):654–8.

91. Declercq ER, Sakala C, Corry MP, et al. Listening to Mothers II: report of the Second National U.S. Survey of Women's Childbearing Experiences. New York: Childbirth Connection; 2006.

92. Melnikow J, Romano P, Gilbert WM, et al. Vaginal birth after cesarean in California. Obstet Gynecol 2001;98:421–6.

93. Little MO, Lyerly AD, Mitchell LM, et al. Mode of delivery: toward responsible inclusion of patient preferences. Obstet Gynecol 2008;112(4):913–8.

94. Guise JM. A guest editorial: the ethics of childbirth: are all roads leading to cesarean? Obstet Gynecol Surv 2001;56(10):593–5.

95. Deering SH, Zaret J, McGaha K, et al. Patients presenting with birth plans: a case control study of delivery outcomes. J Reprod Med 2007;52:884–7.

96. Pang MW, Law LW, Leung TY, et al. Sociodemographic factors and pregnancy events associated with women who declined cesarean section. Eur J Obstet Gynecol Reprod Biol 2009;143(1):24–8.

97. Eden K, Hashima J, Osterweil P. Childbirth preferences after cesarean birth: a review of the evidence. Birth 2004;31:49–60.

98. Lyerly AD, Mitchell LM, Armstrong EM, et al. Risks, values, and decision-making surrounding pregnancy. Obstet Gynecol 2007;109(4):979–84.

99. Harer W. Patient choice cesarean. ACOG Clin Rev 2000;5:1–16.

100. Paterson-Brown S, Fisk NM. Caesarean section: every woman's right to choose? Curr Opin Obstet Gynecol 1997;9:351–5.

101. Moffat MA, Bell JS, Porter MA, et al. Decision making about mode of delivery among pregnant women who have previously had a caesarean section: a qualitative study. BJOG 2007;114(1):86–93.

102. McClain CS. The making of a medical tradition: vaginal birth after cesarean. Soc Sci Med 1990;31(2):203–10.

103. Renner RM, Eden KB, Osterweil P, et al. Informational factors influencing patient's childbirth preferences after prior cesarean. Am J Obstet Gynecol 2007;196(5):e14–6.

104. Eden KB, Dolan JG, Perrin NA, et al. Patients were more consistent in randomized trial at prioritizing childbirth preferences using graphic-numeric than verbal formats. J Clin Epidemiol 2009;62(4):415–24, e413.

105. Montgomery AA, Emmett CL, Fahey T, et al. Two decision aids for mode of delivery among women with previous caesarean section: randomised controlled trial. BMJ 2007;334(7607):1305.

106. Shorten A, Shorten B, Keogh J, et al. Making choices for childbirth: a randomized controlled trial of a decision-aid for informed birth after cesarean. Birth 2005;32(4):252–61.

107. Frost J, Shaw A, Montgomery A, et al. Women's views on the use of decision aids for decision making about the method of delivery following a previous caesarean section: qualitative interview study. BJOG 2009;116(7):896–905.

108. Baker DW. The meaning and measure of health literacy. J Gen Intern Med 2006; 21:878–83.

109. Nielsen-Bohlman L, Panzer AM, Kindig DA, editors. Health literacy: a prescription to end confusion. Washington, DC: The National Academies Press; 2004. p. 345.
110. Berkman ND, DeWalt DA, Pignone MP, et al. Literacy and health outcomes. Agency for Healthcare Research and Quality; 2004. Available at: http://www.ahrq.gov/clinic/tp/littp.htm. Accessed December 1, 2010.
111. Cruikshank DP. Informed consent, patient choice, and physician responsibility [editorial]. Obstet Gynecol 1999;94:142–3.
112. Kolstad JT, Chernew ME. Quality and consumer decision making in the market for health insurance and health care services. Med Care Res Rev 2009;66(1): 28S–52S.
113. Blendon RJ, DesRoches CM, Brodie M, et al. Views of practicing physicians and the public on medical errors. N Engl J Med 2002;347(24):1933–40.
114. Newhouse JP. Why is there a quality chasm? Health Aff 2002;21(4):13–25.
115. Faber M, Bosch M, Wollersheim H, et al. Public reporting in health care: how do consumers use quality-of-care information? A systematic review. Med Care 2009;47(1):1–8.
116. Lothian J. Birth plans: the good, the bad, and the future. J Obstet Gynecol Neonatal Nurs 2006;35:295–303.
117. Lubalin JS, Harris-Kojetin L. What do consumers want and need to know in making health care choices? Med Care Res Rev 1999;56(Suppl 1):67–102.
118. Bernstein AM, Gauthier AK. Choices in healthcare: what are they and what are they worth? Med Care Res Rev 1999;56(Suppl 1):5–23.
119. Phibbs CS, Mark DH, Luft HS, et al. Choice of hospital for delivery: a comparison of high-risk and low-risk women. Health Serv Res 1993;28(2):201–22.
120. Roh CY, Moon M. Nearby, but not wanted? The bypassing of rural hospitals and policy implications for rural health care systems. Policy Stud J 2005;33:477–94.
121. Gaskin DJ, Hadley J, Freeman VG. Are urban safety-net hospitals losing low-risk Medicaid maternity patients? Health Serv Res 2001;36(1 Pt 1):25–51.
122. Taylor SL, Capella LM. Hospital outshopping: determinant attributes and hospital choice. Health Care Manage Rev 1996;21(4):33–44.
123. Gooding SK. The effect of consumer perceptions of quality and sacrifice on hospital choice: a suburban vs. urban competitive scenario. J Hosp Mark 1996;11(1):81–94.
124. Roh C-Y, Lee K-H, Fottler MD. Determinants of hospital choice of rural hospital patients: The impact of networks, service scopes, and market competition. J Med Syst 2008;32:343–53.
125. Luft H, Garnick D, Mark D, et al. Does quality influence choice of hospital? JAMA 1990;263:2899–906.
126. McDaniel C, Gates R, Lamb CW Jr. Who leaves the service area? Profiling the hospital outshopper. J Health Care Mark 1992;12(3):2–9.
127. Weng HC. Consumer empowerment behavior and hospital choice. Health Care Manage Rev 2006;31(3):197–204.
128. Britton JR. Global satisfaction with perinatal hospital care: stability and relationship to anxiety depression, and stressful medical events. Am J Med Qual 2006; 21(3):200–5.
129. Meyer JH. Informed consent, informed refusal, and informed choices. Am J Obstet Gynecol 2003;189:319–26.
130. Wathieu L, Brenner L, Carmon Z, et al. Consumer control and empowerment: a primer. Mark Lett 2002;13(3):297–305.

131. Sofaer S, Crofton C, Goldstein E, et al. What do consumers want to know about the quality of care in hospitals? Health Serv Res 2005;40(6 Part 2):2018–36.
132. Gregory KD, Fridman M, Shah S, et al. Global measures of quality and patient safety related childbirth outcomes: should we monitor adverse or ideal rates? Am J Obstet Gynecol 2009;200(6):681, e1–7.
133. Renkert S, Nutbeam D. Opportunities to improve maternal health literacy through antenatal education: an exploratory study. Health Promot Int 2001; 16(4):381–8.
134. Hall MF, DeFrances CJ, Williams SN, et al. National Hospital Discharge Survey: 2007 summary. Natl Health Stat Report 2010;29:1–24.
135. Cannon CP. Time to treatment of acute myocardial infarction revisited. Curr Opin Cardiol 1998;13(4):254–66.
136. Siassakos D, Hasafa Z, Sibanda T, et al. Retrospective cohort study of diagnosis-delivery interval with umbilical cord prolapse: the effect of team training. BJOG 2009;116:1089–96.
137. Yeast JD, Poskin M, Stockbauer JW, et al. Changing patterns in regionalization of perinatal care and the impact on neonatal mortality. Am J Obstet Gynecol 1998;178(1):131–5.
138. Holmstrom ST, Phibbs CS. Regionalization and mortality in neonatal intensive care. Pediatr Clin North Am 2009;56(3):617–30.
139. Phibbs CS, Baker LC, Caughey AB, et al. Level and volume of neonatal intensive care and mortality in very-low-birth-weight infants. JAMA 2007;356:2165–75.
140. Lasswell SM, Barfield WD, Rochat RW, et al. Perinatal regionalization for very low-birth-weight and very preterm infants. JAMA 2010;304(9):992–1000.
141. Minkoff H, Ecker J. Is there a doctor in the house? Standards of physician availability for laboring women. Obstet Gynecol 2010;116:723–7.
142. Lorenzi NM, Riley RT, Blyth AJC, et al. Antecedents of the people and organizational aspects of medical informatics: review of the literature. JAMA 1997;4(2): 79–93.
143. Shortliffe EH. Strategic action in health information technology: why the obvious has taken so long. Health Aff 2005;24(5):1222–33.
144. Korst LM, Signer JMK, Aydin CE, et al. Identifying organizational capacities and incentives for datasharing: the case of a regional perinatal information system. JAMA 2008;15(2):195–7.

VBAC: A Medicolegal Perspective

Clarissa Bonanno, MD[a],*, Marilee Clausing, RN, BSN, JD[b],
Richard Berkowitz, MD[a]

KEYWORDS

- VBAC • Trial of labor after cesarean • Malpractice
- Medicolegal

History has always been a series of pendulum swings, and there is perhaps no better example in obstetrics than that of vaginal birth after cesarean (VBAC).

The phrase "once a cesarean always a cesarean" was coined by Edward B. Cragin in 1916.[1] Dr Cragin was referring to a very small proportion of pregnant women who were unable to deliver vaginally after several days in active labor and required cesarean delivery as a life-saving procedure. Despite the perils of surgery in that era, these women were not believed to be candidates for vaginal delivery in the future. Although this approach prevailed for more than 5 decades, the overall cesarean rate, and thus the repeat cesarean rate, remained low. When the rate of cesarean delivery in the United States was first measured in 1965, it was 4.5%.[2] During this period, surgery became much safer with the advent of modern surgical techniques, anesthetic agents, antibiotics, and blood transfusion.

The cesarean delivery rate began to rise in the 1970s. Consequently, patients and providers began questioning the paradigm of routine repeat cesarean deliveries. In 1981, a National Institutes of Health (NIH) Consensus Development Conference Panel on Cesarean Childbirth addressed this issue and recommended that more women who had undergone a previous cesarean delivery be offered a trial of labor.[3] The American College of Obstetricians and Gynecologists (ACOG) also concluded that carefully selected patients should be allowed a trial of labor after cesarean in its first publication on VBAC in 1982.[4]

With the advent of managed care in the 1990s, health maintenance organizations and insurers began to promote VBAC as a cost-saving measure; some even went so far as to mandate trial of labor after cesarean (TOLAC) and to withhold reimbursement for elective repeat cesareans. Because of these factors, VBAC rates steadily increased from 19.9% in 1990 to a peak of 28.3% in 1996.[5] Over the same period,

[a] Department of Obstetrics Gynecology, Columbia University, 622 West 168th Street, PH 16-66, New York, NY 10032, USA
[b] Anderson, Rasor & Partners, LLP, 100 South Wacker Drive, Suite 1000, Chicago, IL 60606, USA
* Corresponding author.
E-mail address: cab90@columbia.edu

Clin Perinatol 38 (2011) 217–225
doi:10.1016/j.clp.2011.03.005
0095-5108/11/$ – see front matter © 2011 Elsevier Inc. All rights reserved.

the total cesarean delivery rate declined, from 22.7% to 20.7%, partly because of the decrease in repeat procedures.[5]

What happened next is well-known: the pendulum came back swiftly. VBAC rates declined dramatically over the next decade, to a low of 8.5% in 2006.[6] The cesarean delivery rate, meanwhile, has continued to rise unabated with the most recent estimate for 2008 reaching 32.3%.[7]

Several explanations have been ascribed to these trends. A landmark study published in the New England Journal of Medicine in 1996 by McMahon and colleagues[8] reported that major maternal complications were nearly twice as likely among women attempting a TOLAC compared with those who underwent an elective repeat cesarean. As more reports on adverse outcomes appeared after the McMahon article, liability pressure over the issue of VBAC grew. In response to this issue, ACOG revised its statement on VBAC in 1999, changing the tone of its language considerably.[9,10] Although the previous statement had encouraged a TOLAC for all women without contraindications, the new bulletin stated that women without contraindications should be "offered" a trial of labor. Even more importantly, they recommended that physicians and resources for emergency cesareans be "immediately available" to these patients. Unable to comply with these recommendations or unwilling to incur the risk of litigation, many physicians and hospitals across the country stopped offering TOLACs, limiting patient access to this option. In fact, approximately one-third of hospitals and one-half of physicians are no longer offering women a TOLAC.[11]

This past year, the NIH convened a Consensus Development Conference focused on the issue of VBAC.[11] The hope of the conference was that an updated review of the relevant literature would help inform the decisions made by both patients and providers when considering mode of delivery after cesarean. The panel specifically recommended that ACOG and the American Society of Anesthesiologists reassess the "immediately available" requirement, citing the low level of evidence for this recommendation and the limited access to trial of labor for women that has resulted. ACOG subsequently qualified but did not rescind the "immediately available" requirement.[12] Only time will tell the long-term effect of the conference on VBAC and cesarean rates, and ultimately where the pendulum will come to rest.

What are the fundamental reasons why many hospitals and physicians are no longer performing VBACs? The answer is undoubtedly risk of adverse outcomes and subsequent litigation. The recent NIH Consensus Conference Statement on VBAC acknowledged that the "current medical-legal environment—including provider perceptions of and experience with professional liability—exerts a chilling effect on the availability of trial of labor."[11] Perhaps an exploration of each of the medical and legal risks will shed light on this contentious issue.

As James R. Scott, MD,[13] aptly put in his editorial for the recent conference publication, "VBAC is essentially a uterine rupture issue." The greatest morbidity from TOLAC for mothers and infants clearly arises from uterine rupture. According to the recent conference statement, the risk of uterine rupture for women who undergo a trial of labor at term is 778 per 100,000 (0.778%), compared with 22 per 100,000 (0.00022%) for women who undergo a repeat cesarean at term.[11] Although several groups have tried to develop prediction models, no reliable method currently exists to predict which patients will experience a uterine rupture.[14,15] Even the factors commonly understood to increase the risk of uterine rupture, such as classical and low vertical uterine incisions, increasing number of prior cesarean deliveries, and induction of labor, are based on low-grade evidence according to the consensus panel.[11]

For patients who have a uterine rupture, what is the likelihood of neonatal death or neurologic injury? Approximately 6% of all uterine ruptures will result in perinatal death, and for term pregnancies the risk is less than 3%.[11] Unfortunately, data on the risk of hypoxic ischemic encephalopathy (HIE) after uterine rupture are limited, and scant information is available on the overall rate of long-term adverse neurologic outcome. In the large, prospective observational study of 33,699 women with prior cesarean conducted by the Maternal-Fetal Medicine Units Network, the incidence of HIE was significantly higher with trial of labor (12 cases) than repeat cesarean (0 cases).[16] The absolute risk of HIE after uterine rupture in this study was 0.46 per 1000.

Evidence shows that the incidence of uterine rupture may be higher in the community hospital setting.[17] In addition, a large retrospective cohort study from Scotland showed that the risk of perinatal death from uterine rupture was significantly greater in hospitals with less than 3000 births per year compared with those with 3000 or more births per year.[18] The authors concluded that the resources available at larger obstetric units may reduce the risk of perinatal death at these centers.

Certainly the risk of uterine rupture, and consequently the delivery of a neonate who dies or experiences permanent neurologic sequelae, seem to be low. Conservatively, if 1% of patients attempting a TOLAC have a uterine rupture, and 10% of those infants experience irrevocable damage, that risk is approximately 1 in 1000 TOLACs. This risk is on the order of other invasive procedures performed in pregnancy, and even lower than other diagnostic procedures such as amniocentesis and chorionic villus sampling (CVS), which may lead to pregnancy loss.

Of course, providers and hospitals must also contend with legal risk when deciding whether to offer TOLAC. No comprehensive data are available on the reasons for malpractice suits in VBAC cases. However, the primary reason for litigation in obstetrics is the neurologically compromised child, which seems to hold true for VBAC cases. A major difference from the non–VBAC-related cases of neurologically impaired infants is that the proximate cause for the adverse neurologic outcome in most VBAC cases is generally uterine rupture.

The cost of caring for children with severe neurologic impairment is tremendous, which translates into significant potential damages in malpractice cases. The median award by jury verdict for "medical negligence in childbirth cases" has reached $2.3 million.[19] As a result, obstetricians pay upwards of $200,000 per year in malpractice insurance in some states, with an estimated 60% of these premiums going toward lawsuits for cerebral palsy allegedly caused by birth injury.[20] Unfortunately, liability insurers are motivated to settle cases in which the potential damages are high, regardless of the merit of the claim. What is the bottom line for providers of TOLAC? They could potentially be involved in a lawsuit in which a large settlement is paid, even if the standard of care was met.

ACOG members have confirmed that liability concerns have influenced their practice patterns. According to the 2009 ACOG Survey on Professional Liability, 25.9% of members stopped offering TOLAC services over the previous 3 years.[21] In a separate question, 19.5% of respondents reported that they stopped offering TOLACs because of malpractice insurance affordability or availability. Litigation is more than a theoretical concern for members; 90.5% of respondents had experienced at least one professional liability claim during their professional careers, with an average of 2.69 claims per member. Although survey results may be influenced by response bias, other studies have confirmed that higher malpractice premiums are associated with higher cesarean rates and lower rates of VBAC.[22] In one analysis, the authors estimated that a $10,000 decrease in malpractice premiums for obstetrician-gynecologists would translate into approximately 6000 fewer cesareans and 1600 more VBACs.[22] Rising malpractice premiums also seem to be associated with an increased rate of exit and a reduced rate of entry for obstetricians in certain states.[23]

What are the critical liability issues for obstetricians providing VBAC today? Since the 1999 ACOG bulletin on VBAC, the standard of care according to the College dictated that TOLAC should be attempted in institutions equipped to respond to emergencies with physicians "immediately available." This standard is problematic for numerous reasons.

The definition of "immediately available" is obscure. ACOG may have intended to have individual hospitals decide how to define "immediately available." The implication, of course, is that these physicians will be able to respond to an emergency such as a uterine rupture faster than a physician who is "readily available" and thereby avert disaster. But how fast must the response be? In its 2007 Guidelines for Perinatal Care, the ACOG suggested that any hospital providing obstetric service should have the capability of responding to an obstetric emergency.[24] Specifically, the document states that "in general, the consensus has been that hospitals should have the capability of beginning a cesarean within 30 minutes of the decision to operate."

In cases of uterine rupture, however, 30 minutes may not be fast enough. In a retrospective review of 106 cases of uterine rupture, significant neonatal morbidity occurred when more than 18 minutes elapsed between the onset of a prolonged deceleration and delivery.[25] A smaller subsequent study showed that even this threshold did not universally prevent severe acidosis and morbidity, perhaps because of the confounding factors of placental or fetal extrusion.[26] The guidelines do cite uterine rupture, cord prolapse, placental abruption, and hemorrhage from placenta previa as examples in which the delivery may need to be "more expeditious" than 30 minutes, without further specification.[24] However, a decision-to-delivery time of even 30 minutes may not be achievable in all labor suites across the country. Clearly too few anesthesia providers or operating rooms are available to ensure "immediately available" operative services in all labor suites.[11] Although it may be more feasible to have obstetric providers immediately available for patients attempting VBAC, resources for emergency cesareans even in tertiary care centers are not unlimited and are affected by patient volume, acuity, and manpower.

Given that the perinatal morbidity and mortality rates associated with TOLAC are similar to those of any nulligravid patient in labor, why is TOLAC held to a higher standard? Is it because TOLAC is still viewed as an elective procedure with risks that could be avoided by a repeat cesarean? Or is this simply the first example of more rigorous guidelines to come for the management of all obstetric emergencies?

In the most recent Practice Bulletin on VBAC published in August of this year, ACOG upholds its "immediately available" recommendation, but goes on to say that "when resources for immediate cesarean delivery are not available... providers and patients considering TOLAC discuss the hospital's resources and availability of obstetric, pediatric, anesthetic and operating room staffs."[12] Furthermore, the "decision to offer and pursue TOLAC in a setting in which the option of immediate cesarean delivery is more limited should be carefully considered by patients and their health care providers."[12]

Clearly the College recognizes that the "immediately available" recommendation is not feasible in many hospitals throughout the country. Rather than infringe on patient autonomy by mandating repeat cesareans in these circumstances, ACOG is trying to support the option for women to make an informed decision to accept this increased level of risk. However, this caveat will do nothing to change the current climate of VBAC in the United States. Who is responsible for determining which labor suites could have had providers immediately available for an emergency? Providers are already abandoning the practice of VBAC in sizable numbers because of litigation risk. They will unlikely be willing to assume an increased level of risk, even if their patients are willing to do so.

Patients make decisions based on their perceptions of risk on a regular basis, after being informed by their providers about the consequences of their choices. Some of these decisions will involve potential risk to the fetus or child. Will I have an amniocentesis? Will I take this medication for my seizure disorder? Will I undergo a trial of labor? Physicians also have to make decisions about which procedures to offer patients based on training, experience, and risk, including risk of a lawsuit. A TOLAC is essentially an elective procedure, and undoubtedly a physician can lose a major lawsuit even when a uterine rupture is managed perfectly. Is it wrong then, for some physicians and hospitals to consider that risk unacceptable?

How can physicians protect themselves from liability in TOLAC cases? A pristine informed consent process, combined with pristine management by the obstetric care providers, and documentation of both, is the optimal situation for success in the courtroom. Because the proximate cause of the adverse neurologic outcome is generally known (ie, uterine rupture), there is rarely an effective alternative "causation defense" to the injury. Therefore, to maximize defensibility of the case, the standard of care for managing patients undergoing TOLAC should be strictly followed.

First, informed consent must be properly obtained. Informed consent is a process of communication between a patient and physician that should precede the patient's decision regarding a specific medical intervention. Simply asking a patient to sign a consent form, no matter how broad or detailed, does not constitute informed consent. The standard components of any informed consent process should include discussion and documentation of (1) the patient's diagnosis, (2) the nature and purpose of the proposed intervention, (3) the risks and benefits of the proposed intervention, (4) alternative interventions and their risks and benefits, and (5) the risks of not undergoing any or all interventions. The authors' suggestions for items to be included in the ideal consent form for TOLAC are listed in **Box 1**.

Several points are critical to the discussion of TOLAC versus elective repeat cesarean. First, the risks and benefits of each option must relate to the patient, her fetus/neonate, and her potential future pregnancies. The discussion should be tailored to individual factors that will influence the patient's success rate (eg, age, parity, body mass index, indication for previous cesarean, history of vaginal delivery, gestational age, estimated fetal weight, need for induction). When possible, this discussion should begin early in the antenatal period and be revisited as circumstances arise during the prenatal course that will influence the patient's risks and/or benefits. The process continues throughout the labor course as the status of labor progress becomes evident.

Warning signs for uterine rupture are listed in **Box 2**. Continuation of a trial of labor in the setting of these signs is inadvisable. However, the decision to continue with a TOLAC should be reviewed in the setting of poor labor progress when whether to augment labor with pitocin must be determined. Patients should be made aware of their right to revoke consent for TOLAC at any time during labor and opt for a cesarean. Even in the absence of any obstetric or medical indication to undergo repeat cesarean, continuing with TOLAC after the patient has requested a cesarean is considered proceeding without consent.[27]

Second, physicians must practice evidence-based medicine, including following the generally accepted standards of labor progress in the active phase. They must adhere to the guidelines for oxytocin use at their institution. The standard nomenclature must be used for the classification and interpretation of fetal heart rate tracings. Although these recommendations may seem obvious, many VBAC lawsuits hinge on alleged inappropriate use of oxytocin, failure to interpret the fetal heart rate tracing properly, or failure to perform a timely cesarean.

Box 1
Suggested elements of informed consent for TOLAC

- The patient understands her options of either undergoing a repeat cesarean delivery or TOLAC
- The risks and benefits of each of these options are discussed with the patient
- The success rate of VBAC is between 60% and 80%
- Factors for each patient that will either increase or decrease her expected success rate are noted in the discussion
  - Increased success: prior vaginal delivery, prior VBAC, spontaneous labor, prior cesarean for a nonrecurrent indication (eg, breech presentation)
  - Decreased success: advanced maternal age, non-white ethnicity, maternal obesity, recurrent indication for the prior cesarean, higher estimated fetal weight/suspected macrosomia, gestational age >40 weeks, need for induction of labor
- The risk of uterine rupture is 0.5% to 1% for patients with one prior low transverse cesarean delivery
- Some literature supports an increased risk of uterine rupture In the setting of induction or augmentation of labor, and suggests the risk may increase with higher dosages of pitocin
  - The patient may attempt a TOLAC but decline use of induction/augmentation agents
- A failed TOLAC is associated with a higher risk of complications than an elective repeat cesarean, because most maternal morbidity occurs when a cesarean becomes necessary during labor and/or a uterine rupture occurs
- A ruptured uterus may result in maternal complications such as hemorrhage, organ injury, infection, thromboembolism, hysterectomy, brain damage, and death
- A ruptured uterus may result in severe neonatal complications, including brain damage and/or death
- If the uterus ruptures, insufficient time may be available to operate and prevent permanent injury to or death of the infant, even under the most optimal circumstances
- The hospital's resources, including the availability of obstetric, pediatric, anesthetic, and operating room staff, are reviewed
- At any point before or during the labor course the patient may revoke her consent for TOLAC and proceed with a repeat cesarean

These are the authors' suggestions for the elements of the ideal informed consent process and should not be considered the current standard of care for the management of these patients.

Finally, everything must be documented. The informed consent process should be documented in the patient's medical record wherever appropriate. The patient's signature at the bottom of a standard Labor and Delivery consent form does not suffice. Physicians are advised to have the patient sign a specific consent form for TOLAC during the antenatal period, and this form should be referenced or reaffirmed when she is admitted to the labor unit. In addition, discussions and decisions made during the course of labor should be documented thoroughly.

How protective will these efforts be? In the setting of adequate informed consent, in which the standard of care was met for the management of a patient undergoing TOLAC, and for which all events were sufficiently documented in the medical record, will providers still be subject to successful lawsuits? Unfortunately, the answer is yes. A 1996 study of malpractice cases showed that the severity of the patient's disability was predictive of payment to the plaintiff, whereas the occurrence of an adverse event

---

Box 2
Warning signs of uterine rupture

- Fetal heart rate tracing abnormalities
  - Classic pattern: recurrent variable decelerations
  - Other patterns: bradycardia, recurrent late decelerations
- Severe, acute, constant abdominal pain
- Loss of fetal station
- Heavy vaginal bleeding
- Maternal tachycardia and/or hypotension

---

related to negligence was not. This is probably because the former cases were preferentially settled rather than risk an exorbitant jury verdict.[28] However, rigorous informed consent and standard of care management should maximize protection for physicians offering TOLAC.

In another analysis of claims involving obstetric practice, Clark and colleagues[29] found that 80% of cases involving VBAC were avoidable had three conditions been met: (1) trials were limited to women entering labor spontaneously, (2) trials continued only if a normal, nonaugmented labor curve was followed, (3) trials continued only in the absence of significant, repetitive variable decelerations or other indicators of fetal compromise. Although this strategy may be more protective from litigation, it would significantly restrict the number of candidates for this procedure, and likely reduce the number who will have a successful VBAC. Can restricting trials of VBAC in the interest of preventing litigation be justified? Or could an approach like this be a compromise for lower-resource settings in which TOLAC is not likely to be available at all?

Regionalization of care has also been proposed as a mechanism to facilitate access for patients desiring TOLAC. Although this may be feasible for urban areas with multiple large medical centers, the need is greatest in rural settings where the logistics of this strategy would be formidable. The notion of individual centers developing expertise in managing TOLACs has definite appeal, which may translate into improved outcomes for these patients. However, this model does not address the increased litigation risk that these centers might face.

The ultimate solution to the VBAC dilemma will clearly not be found within the current system. Medical courts, tighter regulation of medical experts, dispute resolution, and no-fault regulation have all been described as potential ways to make the system more efficient, more equitable, and ultimately more supportive of families who need financial support regardless of whether the injury was a result of medical negligence.[30] In addition, more concerted efforts to enhance patient safety should offset some of the pressure of liability.[31]

In his Inaugural Address from the 2010 Annual Meeting as the new President of ACOG, Dr Richard N. Waldman stated:

Each one of us enters the labor and delivery room shouldering our concern for our two patients and weighed down by the overwhelming yoke of liability. Our decisions are still made as much by art as they are by science. We have always accepted the burden of making the difficult decisions for mother and baby but they were hard enough before the culture of legal fear invaded our maternity units. Those buck stop here decisions are tough enough without fears of losing our liability insurance, our livelihood, our financial reserves, or being publicly humiliated. Liability dampens our spirits but unfortunately, it is also starting to define our specialty.[32]

The hope is that in the coming years liability concerns will not result in an end to the practice of VBAC.

REFERENCES

1. Cragin EB. Conservatism in obstetrics. NY Med J 1916;104:1–3.
2. Taffel SM, Placek PJ, Liss T. Trends in the United States cesarean section rate and reasons for the 1980–1985 rise. Am J Public Health 1987;77:955–9.
3. National Institutes of Health. Consensus development conference on cesarean childbirth. Washington, DC: NIH; 1981. Pub. No. 82:2067.
4. American College of Obstetrician Gynecologists. Committee statement guidelines for vaginal delivery after cesarean childbirth. Washington, DC: ACOG; 1982.
5. Menacker F. Trends in cesarean rates for first births and repeat cesarean rates for low-risk women: United States, 1990–2003. Natl Vital Stat Rep 2005;54(4):1–8.
6. Martin JA, Hamilton BE, Sutton PD, et al. Births: final data for 2006. Natl Vital Stat Rep 2009;57(7):1–104.
7. Hamilton BE, Martin JA, Ventura SJ. Births: preliminary data for 2008. Natl Vital Stat Rep 2010;58(16):1–13.
8. McMahon MJ, Luther ER, Bowes WA, et al. Comparison of a trial of labor with an elective second cesarean section. N Engl J Med 1996;335:689–95.
9. American College of Obstetricians and Gynecologists (ACOG). Vaginal delivery after a cesarean birth. Practice Patterns No 1. Washington, DC: ACOG; 1995.
10. American College of Obstetricians and Gynecologists (ACOG). Vaginal birth after previous cesarean delivery. ACOG Practice Bulletin No 5. Washington, DC: ACOG; 1999. p. 1106–12.
11. NIH Conference Statement. Vaginal birth after cesarean. Obstet Gynecol 2010; 115:1279–95.
12. American College of Obstetricians and Gynecologists (ACOG). Vaginal birth after previous cesarean delivery. ACOG Practice Bulletin No 115. Washington, DC: ACOG; 2010.
13. Scott JR. Solving the vaginal birth after cesarean dilemma. Obstet Gynecol 2010; 116:1112–3.
14. Macones GA, Cahill AG, Stamilio DM, et al. Can uterine rupture in patients attempting vaginal delivery be predicted? Am J Obstet Gynecol 2006;195: 1148–52.
15. Grobman WA, Lai Y, Landon MB, et al. Prediction of uterine rupture associated with attempted vaginal delivery vaginal birth after cesarean delivery. Am J Obstet Gynecol 2008;199:e1–30. e5.
16. Landon MB, Hauth JC, Leveno KJ, et al. Maternal and perinatal outcomes associated with a trial of labor after prior cesarean delivery. N Engl J Med 2004;351: 2581–9.
17. Blanchette H, Blanchette M, McCabe J, et al. Is vaginal birth after cesarean safe? Experience at a community hospital. Am J Obstet Gynecol 2001;184:1478–87.
18. Smith GCS, Pell JP, Pasupathy D, et al. Factors predisposing to perinatal death related to uterine rupture during attempted vaginal birth after cesarean section: retrospective cohort study. BMJ 2004;329:375–9.
19. Rybak EA. Hippocratic ideal, Faustian bargain and Damocles' sword: erosion of patient autonomy in obstetrics. J Perinatol 2009;29:721–5.

20. Freeman JM, Freeman AD. No-fault neurological compensation: perhaps its time has come, again. Harvard Med Instit Forum 2003;23:5–6.
21. American College of Obstetrician Gynecologists. ACOG survey on professional liability. Washington, DC: American College of Obstetrician Gynecologists; 2009.
22. Yang YT, Mello MM, Subramanian SV, et al. Relationship between malpractice litigation pressure and rates of cesarean section and vaginal birth after cesarean section. Med Care 2009;47:234–42.
23. Polsky D, Marcus SC, Werner RM. Malpractice premiums and the supply of obstetricians. Inquiry 2010;47:48–61.
24. American College of Obstetricians and Gynecologists (ACOG), American Academy of Pediatrics (AAP). Guidelines for perinatal care. 6th edition. Washington, DC: American College of Obstetricians and Gynecologists; 2007. p. 159.
25. Leung A, Leung EK, Paul RH. Uterine rupture after previous cesarean delivery: maternal and fetal consequences. Am J Obstet Gynecol 1993;169:945–50.
26. Bujold E, Gauthier R. Neonatal morbidity associated with uterine rupture: what are the risk factors? Am J Obstet Gynecol 2002;186:311–4.
27. Phelan JP. Time to reconsider? OBG Management 1996;11:62–8.
28. Brennan TA, Cox CM, Burstin HR. Relation between negligent adverse events and the outcomes of medical-malpractice litigation. N Engl J Med 1996;335: 1963–7.
29. Clark AL, Belfort MA, Dildy GA, et al. Reducing obstetric litigation through alterations in practice patterns. Obstet Gynecol 2008;112:1279–83.
30. Hankins GD, MacLennan AH, Speer ME, et al. Obstetric litigation is asphyxiating our maternity services. Obstet Gynecol 2006;107:1382–5.
31. Abuhamad A, Grobman WA. Patient safety and medical liability. Obstet Gynecol 2010;116:570–7.
32. Waldman RN. Together we can do something wonderful. Obstet Gynecol 2010; 115:1116–9.

An Ethical Framework for the Informed Consent Process for Trial of Labor After Cesarean Delivery

Frank A. Chervenak, MD[a],*, Laurence B. McCullough, PhD[b]

KEYWORDS

• Informed consent • VBAC • Cesearean delivery • TOLAC

In 2010, an important year for the topic of vaginal birth after cesarean delivery (VBAC), both a National Institutes of Health (NIH) consensus panel,[1] on which one of the authors (LBM) served, and the American College of Obstetricians and Gynecologists (ACOG)[2] issued updated statements. Both statements agree that there should be a thorough, evidence-based informed consent process in which pregnant women with a prior cesarean delivery are counseled concerning the option of VBAC. The evidence base for this counseling is discussed elsewhere in this issue. Both statements also agree that ethics is an essential dimension of counseling about VBAC. The purpose of this article is to provide a practical ethical framework for physicians to use in the informed consent process for trial of labor after cesarean delivery (TOLAC).

A PRIMER ON OBSTETRIC ETHICS

Ethics has been understood for centuries in the history of philosophy as the disciplined study of morality. Medical ethics is the disciplined study of morality in medicine. On the basis of reasoned argument, medical ethics seeks to identify in a practical fashion the obligations of physicians and health care organizations to patients as well as the obligations of patients.[3] Medical ethics since the eighteenth-century European and American Enlightenments has been secular in two important senses.[4] It makes no reference to God or revealed tradition but to what reasoned argument requires and produces. At the same time, secular medical ethics is not intrinsically hostile to religious beliefs.

a Department of Obstetrics and Gynecology, New York-Presbyterian Hospital – Weill Cornell Medical College, 525 East 68th Street, M-724, Box 122, New York, NY 10065, USA
b Center for Medical Ethics and Health Policy, Baylor College of Medicine, One Baylor Plaza MS 420, Houston, TX 77030, USA
* Corresponding author.
E-mail address: fac2001@med.cornell.edu

Clin Perinatol 38 (2011) 227–231
doi:10.1016/j.clp.2011.03.002
0095-5108/11/$ – see front matter © 2011 Elsevier Inc. All rights reserved.

Therefore, ethical principles and virtues should be understood to apply to all physicians, regardless of their personal religious and spiritual beliefs.[5]

The traditions and practices of medicine constitute a crucial source of morality for physicians. The traditions and practices of medicine provide an important reference point for medical ethics because they are based on the obligation to protect and promote the health-related interests of patients. This obligation tells physicians what morality in medicine ought to be but in general, abstract terms. Providing a more concrete, clinically applicable account of that obligation is the central task of medical ethics, using the ethical principles of beneficence and respect for autonomy.[3]

The ethical principle of beneficence in general requires one to act in a way that is expected reliably to produce the greater balance of benefits over harms in the lives of others.[5] To put this principle into clinical practice requires a reliable account of the benefits and harms relevant to the care of patients and of how those goods and harms should be reasonably balanced against each other,[6] as is the case for TOLAC. In medicine, the principle of beneficence requires physicians to act in a way that is reliably expected to produce the greater balance of clinical benefits over harms for patients.[3]

Nonmaleficence means that physicians should prevent causing harm and is best understood as expressing the limits of beneficence.[5] This is also known as *primum non nocere* (first do no harm). This commonly invoked dogma is really a latinized misinterpretation of the hippocratic texts, which emphasized beneficence while avoiding harm when approaching the limits of medicine.[3] Nonmaleficence should be incorporated into beneficence-based clinical judgment: when a physician approaches the limits of beneficence-based clinical judgment (ie, when the evidence for expected benefit diminishes and the risks of clinical harm increase), then the physician should proceed with great caution. Physicians should be especially concerned with preventing serious, far-reaching, and irreversible clinical harm to patients.

The ethical principle of respect for patient autonomy requires that physicians always acknowledge and carry out the value-based preferences of adult, competent patients, unless there is compelling ethical justification for not doing so.[5] Pregnant patients increasingly bring to their medical care their own perspective on what is their interest. The principle of respect for autonomy translates into autonomy-based clinical judgment. Because each patient's perspective on her interests is a function of her values and beliefs, it is impossible to specify the benefits and harms of autonomy-based clinical judgment in advance. Indeed, it is inappropriate for a physician to do so, because the definition of her benefits and harms and their balancing are the prerogative of the patient.[3]

The ethical principles of respect for autonomy and beneficence shape the informed consent process.[3,5] We start with the physician's role in that process. Physicians should (1) recognize the capacity of each pregnant patient to deal with medical information and not underestimate that capacity; (2) recognize the validity of the values and beliefs of patients; (3) offer all medically reasonable alternatives for managing a patient's pregnancy (ie, technically possible alternatives supported by evidence-based and beneficence-based clinical judgment about maternal and fetal outcomes); (4) provide information about the clinical benefits and risks of each medically reasonable alternative; (5) recommend a medically reasonable alternative when, in evidence-based clinical judgment, it is clearly superior; (6) recommend against technically possible alternatives that are not supported in evidence-based, beneficence-based clinical judgment; (6) ensure that a patient's decision-making process is voluntary, an especially important consideration regarding pregnant teens; and (7) elicit a patient's value-based preference.[3]

Patients have an important role to play in the informed consent process. Patients should (1) absorb, retain, and recall as needed information about their pregnancy and the medically reasonable alternatives for managing the pregnancy; (2) understand this information; (3) appreciate that this information applies to them; (4) evaluate the medically reasonable alternatives on the basis of their own values and beliefs; and (5) express a value-based preference.[7]

The legal obligations of physicians regarding informed consent were established in a series of cases during the twentieth century. In 1914, *Schloendorff v The Society of The New York Hospital* established the concept of simple consent: Did the patient say "yes" or "no" to medical intervention?[8,9] To this day in the medical and bioethics literature, this decision is quoted: "Every human being of adult years and sound mind has the right to determine what shall be done with his body, and a surgeon who performs an operation without his patient's consent commits an assault for which he is liable in damages."[9] The legal requirement of consent further evolved to include disclosure of information sufficient to enable patients to make informed decisions about whether to say "yes" or "no" to medical intervention.[8]

The ethical principles of beneficence and respect for autonomy play a crucial role in obstetric ethics. There are beneficence-based and autonomy-based obligations to pregnant patients: a physician's perspective on a pregnant woman's health-related interests provides the basis for the physician's beneficence-based obligations to her whereas her own perspective on those interests provides the basis for the physician's autonomy-based obligations to her. Because of an insufficiently developed central nervous system, the fetus cannot meaningfully be said to possess values and beliefs. Thus, there is no basis for saying that a fetus has a perspective on its interests. There can, therefore, be no autonomy-based obligations to any fetus. Hence, the language of fetal rights has no meaning and, therefore, no application to the fetus in obstetric clinical judgment and practice despite its popularity in public and political discourse in the United States and other countries. Physicians have a perspective on a fetus' health-related interests, and physicians can have beneficence-based obligations to a fetus but only when a fetus is a patient.[3]

Rights are not required to be a patient. Rather, being a patient means that a patient can benefit from the applications of the clinical skills of a physician. Put more precisely, a human being without independent moral status is properly regarded as a patient when two conditions are met—that a human being (1) is presented to a physician and (2) there exist clinical interventions that are reliably expected to be efficacious in that they are reliably expected to result in a greater balance of clinical benefits over harms for the human being in question.[3]

The authors have argued elsewhere that beneficence-based obligations to the fetus exist when a fetus is reliably expected later to achieve independent moral status as a child and person.[3] That is, the fetus is a patient when the fetus is presented for medical interventions, whether diagnostic or therapeutic, that reasonably can be expected to result in a greater balance of goods over harms for the child and person the fetus can later become during early childhood. The ethical significance of the concept of the fetus as patient, therefore, depends on links that can be established between the fetus and its later achieving independent moral status.

One such link is viability. Viability, however, must be understood in terms of both biologic and technological factors. It is only by virtue of both factors that a viable fetus can exist ex utero and thus achieve independent moral status. When a fetus is viable, that is, when it is of sufficient maturity so that it can survive into the neonatal period and achieve independent moral status given the availability of the requisite technological support, and when it is presented to the physician, the fetus is a patient.

Viability exists as a function of biomedical and technological capacities, which are different in different parts of the world. As a consequence, there is, at the present time, no worldwide, uniform gestational age to define viability. In the United States, viability presently occurs at approximately 24 weeks of gestational age.[10,11]

The only possible link between a previable fetus and the child it can become is the pregnant woman's autonomy. This is because technological factors cannot result in a previable fetus becoming a child. The link, therefore, between a fetus and the child it can become when the fetus is previable can be established only by the pregnant woman's decision to confer the status of being a patient on her previable fetus. The previable fetus, therefore, has no claim to the status of being a patient independently of the pregnant woman's autonomy. The pregnant woman is free to withhold, confer, or, having once conferred, withdraw the status of being a patient on or from her previable fetus according to her own values and beliefs. The previable fetus is presented to the physician as a function of the pregnant woman's autonomy.[3]

OFFERING AND RECOMMENDING TOLAC IN THE INFORMED CONSENT PROCESS

In some cases, both elective repeat cesarean and TOLAC are supported in evidence-based, beneficence-based clinical judgment and, therefore, should be offered in clinical settings where TOLAC can be performed safely. The NIH consensus panel[1] and ACOG[2] statements agree that TOLAC after a previous single low transverse uterine incision is medically reasonable and should be offered when there was one previous low transverse incision. In the language of obstetric ethics, the evidence supports the clinical judgment that the clinical risks of TOLAC to both pregnant and fetal patients are acceptable when there has been one previous low transverse incision. Elective repeat cesarean delivery also has acceptable risks to both pregnant and fetal patients. Both TOLAC and elective repeat cesarean delivery are, therefore, supported in evidence-based, beneficence-based clinical judgment. Both, therefore, should be offered to pregnant women who have had one previous low transverse incision.

There are some cases in which elective repeat cesarean delivery is substantively supported and TOLAC is not supported in beneficence-based clinical judgment. For example, when a pregnant woman has had a previous classical incision on her uterus, cesarean delivery is preferable to TOLAC because cesarean prevents the fetal and maternal risk of a ruptured classical incision in the uterus. Vaginal delivery in such circumstances results in a substantial increase in morbidity and mortality for both pregnant and fetal patients. Only cesarean delivery should be offered and recommended to pregnant women with a previous classical incision. It follows that obstetricians should recommend against TOLAC in such cases.

TOLAC after to previous low transverse incisions is controversial. The ACOG statement, on the basis of level B evidence, states: "Women with two previous low transverse incisions may be considered candidates for TOLAC."[2] The NIH consensus panel was silent on this topic.[1] Level B evidence is inherently controversial. As a result, competing evidence-based, beneficence clinical judgment about the safety for pregnant and fetal patients of TOLAC when a pregnant woman has had two previous low transverse incisions it to be expected. TOLAC may be offered but an obstetrician is obligated to explain the uncertainties of the evidence.

SUMMARY

Ethics is an essential component of offering and recommending TOLAC in the informed consent process with pregnant women who have had a prior cesarean delivery. For women with one previous low transverse incision, both TOLAC and elective repeat cesarean delivery should be offered. Obstetricians should recommend against TOLAC when pregnant women have had a previous classical incision. TOLAC after two previous low transverse incisions may be offered provided that the informed consent process presents the uncertainties of the evidence.

REFERENCES

1. National Institutes of Health. National Institutes of Health Consensus Development Conference Statement vaginal birth after cesarean: new insights March 8–10, 2010. Semin Perinatol 2010;34:351–65.
2. American College of Obstetricians and Gynecologists. ACOG Practice bulletin no. 115: vaginal birth after prior cesarean delivery. Obstet Gynecol 2010;116(2 Pt 1): 450–63.
3. McCullough LB, Chervenak FA. Ethics in obstetrics and gynecology. New York: Oxford University Press; 1994.
4. Engelhardt HT Jr. The foundations of bioethics. 2nd edition. New York: Oxford University Press; 1995.
5. Beauchamp TL, Childress JF. Principles of biomedical ethics. 6th edition. New York: Oxford University Press; 2009.
6. Chervenak FA, McCullough LB. An ethically justified algorithm for offering, recommending, and performing cesarean delivery and its application in managed care practice. Obstet Gynecol 1996;87:302–5.
7. McCullough LB, Coverdale JH, Chervenak FA. Ethical challenges of decision making with pregnant patients who have schizophrenia. Am J Obstet Gynecol 2002;187:696–702.
8. Faden RR, Beauchamp TL. A history and theory of informed consent. New York: Oxford University Press; 1986.
9. Schloendorff V. The society of the New York Hospital, 211 N.Y. 125, 126, 105 N.E. 92, 93; 1914.
10. Chervenak FA, McCullough LB, Levene MI. An ethically justified clinically comprehensive approach to periviability: gynaecological, obstetric, perinatal, and neonatal dimensions. J Obstet Gynaecol 2007;27:3–7.
11. Skupski DW, Chervenak FA, McCullough LB, et al. Ethical dimensions of periviability. J Perinat Med 2010;38:579–83.

Delivery After Prior Cesarean: Success Rate and Factors

Anthony L. Shanks, MD*, Alison G. Cahill, MD

KEYWORDS

• Vaginal birth after cesarean • Factors • Success
• Prior cesarean • Trial of labor after cesarean

Cesarean delivery rates in the United States have reached an all-time high. The current rate of 31% is 6 times higher than the rate in the 1970s.[1,2] Many factors including physician preference and hospital accessibility account for this trend. A decreased vaginal birth after cesarean (VBAC) rate and an increased repeat cesarean rate have important consequences for women in future pregnancies. Because of these considerations, VBAC has been an important issue within the obstetric community for over 3 decades.

Attempts to decrease the repeat cesarean rate and increase the VBAC rate in the United States resulted in moderate success more than 15 years ago. In 1981, the VBAC rate was 5%. This rate increased to a maximum of 28.3% in 1996.[2,3] Relatively low VBAC rates in the past were likely due to decreased attempts at trial of labor after cesarean (TOLAC) as opposed to actual decreased VBAC success.[4] TOLAC clearly has both short-term and long-term benefits for the women who are successful in achieving a vaginal delivery.[5]

Whereas women who undergo repeat cesarean delivery are subjected to the risks of the surgical procedure—operative injury, blood transfusion, and endometritis—the highest morbidity occurs in women who attempt a TOLAC and are unsuccessful.[6–8] Women who labor and then require cesarean deliveries are subject to the morbidity of the procedure in addition to an exacerbation of the risks inherent in an unscheduled procedure. As the reports of uterine rupture and complications associated with TOLAC have increased, the trend in VBACs over the past decade has shifted in the opposite direction, with a decrease in VBAC rate to 8.5% and a total cesarean rate of 31.1% in 2006.[2]

The current goal of the obstetric community should be to decrease the morbidity in women attempting TOLAC on an individual level as well as to decrease the number of

The authors have no financial disclosures.
Division of Maternal-Fetal Medicine, Department of Obstetrics and Gynecology, Washington University in St Louis, Campus Box 8064, 660 South Euclid, St Louis, MO 63110, USA
* Corresponding author.
E-mail address: shanksa@wudosis.wustl.edu

Clin Perinatol 38 (2011) 233–245
doi:10.1016/j.clp.2011.03.011
0095-5108/11/$ – see front matter © 2011 Elsevier Inc. All rights reserved.

repeat cesarean deliveries. Further, it is critical for practitioners to realize that for women with a history of a prior low transverse cesarean, the mode of delivery associated with the least maternal morbidity is successful TOLAC. Therefore, identifying appropriate candidates, namely women likely to experience success in undergoing TOLAC, is most important.

THE ACOG PERSPECTIVE

The American College of Obstetrics and Gynecology (ACOG) recently updated recommendations for VBAC and TOLAC (2010). The previous practice bulletin highlighted the risk of uterine rupture for women undergoing a TOLAC. These risks differed depending on the location of the incision on the uterus. For women with one prior low transverse uterine incision, the risk of uterine rupture was less than 1% with a TOLAC.[8] For women with incisions that extend into the contractile portion of the uterus, the risk may be as high as 4% to 9%.[9]

Uterine rupture is a potentially catastrophic outcome, and warrants appropriate attention.[10] It has been associated with an increased risk of neonatal compromise, blood transfusion, and hysterectomy. However, the absolute risk is low after one prior cesarean and is also lower than initially estimated for women with a history of 2 or more cesarean deliveries.[8] In a departure from previous ACOG recommendations, 2 prior cesarean deliveries are no longer a contraindication to TOLAC without a prior vaginal birth, and appropriately reflect the best available data.[11,12]

The focus of the updated practice bulletin is identifying appropriate candidates for TOLAC. Whereas successful VBAC is associated with the lowest risk of maternal morbidity, failed TOLAC attempts with subsequent repeat cesarean delivery are associated with the highest. This outcome is likely because of changes to the normal female reproductive anatomy with labor in addition to the emergent nature of the surgery. Maternal outcomes for cesarean delivery after failed TOLAC are clearly worse than with scheduled repeat cesarean section. Proper identification of appropriate candidates thus helps to increase the VBAC rate while minimizing the morbidity of failed TOLACs. The objective of this review is to highlight the data on obstetric factors and assess their impact on VBAC success.

CONTRAINDICATIONS TO TOLAC

The clinician's goal is to identify candidates who are most likely to achieve a successful VBAC. It is therefore prudent to identify patients in whom a TOLAC is contraindicated. Placenta previa and prior fundal surgery are two conditions that warrant specific attention. As previously noted, the risk of uterine rupture with TOLAC after one prior cesarean delivery is known to be less than 1%.[8] Women with prior fundal surgery—previous uterine incisions that extend into the contractile portions of the uterus—have a higher rate of uterine rupture and are poor candidates for a planned TOLAC.[13] It has also been shown that women with a prior uterine rupture have a high likelihood for recurrent rupture. Case series report a risk of recurrent uterine rupture of 6% for scars that are confined to the lower uterine segment. Repeat rupture rates may be as high as 32% for those that extend to the fundus.[14,15]

While not contraindicated from a vaginal delivery, breech presentation and an estimated fetal weight of greater than 5000 g are two examples in which a repeat cesarean delivery may reduce the morbidity to the patient.[16] The mode of delivery can be reevaluated in certain clinical contexts; however, patients with known contraindications to vaginal delivery are clearly poor TOLAC candidates.

FACTORS

The success rate for VBAC has been described as 60% to 80%,[17,18] and the rate may depend on prognostic factors that are identified by the dutiful obstetrician.[19] Indications for the previous cesarean delivery and labor are just two of the factors that have been evaluated to determine VBAC success rates. Gregory and colleagues[20] used a population-based cohort to determine that low-risk women with no maternal, fetal, or placental complications of pregnancy experienced a 73.6% success rate; this was contrasted with a 50.31% success rate for women with one of these factors.

Algorithms and online calculators exist that incorporate these factors and provide individual risk assessments,[21–23] with varying results. The goal of these risk assessments is to identify the patients most likely to deliver vaginally and thereby decrease the chances that a woman will fail a TOLAC. One decision model favored a trial of labor if the VBAC success rate was 50% or more.[24] The most robust prediction model for success to date has been provided by Grobman and colleagues.[25]

Regardless of the nomogram used, clinical acumen remains important to identifying good TOLAC candidates. **Table 1** lists commonly investigated variables and the resulting VBAC success rate. A thorough evaluation of these multiple factors is essential in the process of patient selection.

Prior Vaginal Birth

One of the greatest predictors of VBAC success is prior vaginal delivery, and specifically prior VBAC. Mercer and colleagues[26] used a prospective multicenter registry to estimate the success rates and risk of VBAC stratified by number of prior cesarean deliveries. These investigators found that the rate of uterine rupture decreased after the first successful VBAC and did not increase with subsequent vaginal deliveries (0.87% risk after VBAC, 0.52% after 5 deliveries). The VBAC success rate also increased with increasing numbers of prior VBACs (63.3%, 87.6%, 90.9%, 90.6%, and 91.6% for 0, 1, 2, 3, and 4). The results of this analysis dispelled the notion that multiple VBACs potentially weakened the lower uterine scar and drove home the positive impact of a prior VBAC.

The Maternal-Fetal Medicine Units (MFMU) Cesarean Registry also served Landon and colleagues[27] as an excellent cohort in evaluating the factors that affect VBAC success. Their 4-year multicenter prospective observational study included 14,529 term pregnancies that underwent TOLAC. VBAC was successful in 10,690 (73.6%). Previous vaginal delivery portended the greatest increased odds ratio (OR) for VBAC success (OR 3.9, 95% confidence interval [CI] 3.6–4.3). Other factors predictive of VBAC success included previous indication not for dystocia (OR 1.7, 95% CI 1.5–1.8), spontaneous labor (OR 1.6, 95% CI 1.5–1.8), birth weight <4000 g (OR 2.0, 95% CI 1.0–2.3), and Caucasian race (OR 1.8, 95% CI 1.6–1.9).

In a retrospective cohort analysis of 6619 patients with a prior vaginal delivery, Cahill and colleagues[28] found that women who underwent a TOLAC were less likely to experience uterine rupture, bladder artery, or artery laceration than were women who underwent a repeat cesarean delivery. In that study, women who underwent TOLAC also had a lower risk for fever and transfusions. Women with a prior vaginal delivery who attempt TOLAC should be counseled that they have an increased VBAC success rate with a low complication rate.

Induction/Augmentation of Labor

Induction of labor in patients with a prior cesarean has been associated with an increased risk of uterine rupture. In 2001 Lydon-Rochelle and colleagues[29] evaluated

Table 1
Commonly investigated variables and VBAC success rate

Year	Authors	Type of Study	Variable Analyzed	Patients Undergoing VBAC	VBAC Success Rate
2010	Dharan et al[45]	Retrospective cohort	Diabetics	127	37% (diabetics) vs 56%
2010	Cahill et al[34]	Retrospective cohort	>3 CS	89	79.8% (3) vs 75.5% (1)
2010	Tahseen and Griffiths[32]	Meta-analysis	>2 CS	4064	71.10%
2009	Grobman et al[55]	Mutivariable modeling	Prenatal information	9616	N/A
2009	Costantine et al[53]	Cohort	Prediction model	502	52.20%
2008	Mercer et al[26]	Retrospective cohort	Success with prior vaginal delivery	13532	63.3% (for first VBAC)
2008	Gregory et al[20]	Cohort	Maternal and fetal complications	41450	73.76% (no risk factors) vs 50.31% (high risk)
2007	Srinivas et al[36]	Retrospective cohort	Maternal age	13706	75% (>35 y old)
2007	Erez et al[37]	Retrospective cohort	Mullerian anomalies	103	61.40%
2006	Peaceman et al[38]	Secondary analysis	Fetal birth weight	7081	3.8% decrease in success for each 100 g increase in birth weight
2006	Kiran et al[56]	Retrospective cohort	Gestational age	1620	60%, OR 6.3 (95% CI 1.9–20.2) for scar rupture after EDD
2006	Tripathi et al[17]	Prospective cohort	Indication for previous CS	81	73%
2006	Kraiem et al[57]	Retrospective cohort	Parity, BMI, fetal presentation	352	76.10%
2006	Hollard et al[48]	Retrospective cohort	Ethnicity	8030	79.3% (Caucasian) vs 70.0% (African American)
2005	Macones et al[12]	Retrospective cohort	2 prior CS vs 1 prior	13617	75.5% (1 prior) vs 74.6% (2 prior)

Year	Author	Study type	Focus	N	Result
2005	Landon et al[27]	Prospective cohort	Multiple	14529	73.60%
2005	Pathadey et al[18]	Retrospective cohort	Induction of labor	81	79%
2005	Juhasz et al[42]	Retrospective cohort	BMI, excessive weight gain	1213	77.20%
2005	Quinones et al[50]	Retrospective cohort	Prematurity	12,463	74% (term) and 82% (preterm)
2004	Durnwald et al[43]	Retrospective cohort	Maternal obesity	510	54.6% (obese) vs 70.5% (normal BMI)
2004	Dodd and Crowther[58]	Meta-analysis	Repeat CS vs planned VBAC	449	No significant differences in morbidity
2003	Mankuta et al[24]	Decision analysis	Maternal/fetal morbidities	N/A	Factored by family size
2003	Carroll et al[44]	Retrospective cohort	Maternal weight	219	81.8% (<200 lb), 57.1% (200–300 lb), 13.3% (>300 lb)
2003	Upadhyaya et al[59]	Retrospective cohort	Maternal complications	413	75%
2002	Spaans et al[35]	Retrospective cohort	Oxytocin use, cervical dilation	214	71.40%
2002	Huang et al[52]	Retrospective cohort	Interpregnancy interval	1516	79% (<19 mo) vs 85.5% (>19 mo)
1998	Nassar et al[60]	Retrospective cohort	Severe preeclampsia	145	31.6% (<28 wk) vs 62.5% (>32 wk)
1997	Holt and Mueller[19]	Retrospective cohort	Labor dystocia in index pregnancy	6470	62%
1997	Boulvain et al[61]	Meta-analysis	Maternal factors in developing	—	69%
1996	Bhal et al[62]	Retrospective cohort	Indication for previous CS	471	78.1% (entire cohort) vs 63.8% (CPD, FTP)
1996	Lovell[63]	Retrospective cohort	Nonrecurring indication	244	80.70%
1994	Miller et al[33]	Retrospective cohort	Success with multiple CS	17332	83% (1 prior CS), 75.3% (2 or more)
2005	Landon et al[27]	Prospective cohort	Prior vaginal delivery	14529	86.6% (prior vaginal delivery) vs 60.9% (no prior vaginal delivery)
2006	Cahill et al[28]	Retrospective cohort	Maternal complications in VBAC vs elective CS	5041	Lower rate of maternal complications with VBAC than elective CS

Abbreviations: BMI, body mass index; CI, confidence interval; CPD, cephalopelvic disproportion; CS, cesarean section; EDD, expected date of delivery; FTP, failure to progress; N/A, data not available; OR, odds ratio; VBAC, vaginal birth after cesarean.

20,095 women with a prior cesarean delivery and determined that the risk of rupture was 0.52% if labor occurred spontaneously. This result contrasted with a risk of uterine rupture of 0.77% if labor was induced without prostaglandins and 2.24% if induced with prostaglandins.

Not only is induced labor associated with an increased risk of uterine rupture, it is also less likely to result in successful VBAC.[27,30] In a prospective, observational study of 236 women with a prior cesarean delivery who underwent TOLAC, the vaginal delivery rate was significantly higher in patients who presented in spontaneous labor compared with patients requiring induction (77.1% vs 57.9%, OR 2.45, 95% CI 1.24–4.82).[30] The MFMU study revealed that induction of labor (OR 0.5, 95% CI 0.45–0.55) and augmentation of labor (OR 0.68, 95% CI 0.62–0.75) were both associated with decreased odds of delivering vaginally compared with spontaneous labor.[27]

Conversely, spontaneous labor increases the odds of achieving a successful VBAC. Meta-analyses have consistently shown that spontaneous labor portends a greater chance of VBAC success than induction or augmentation of labor.[31] Although induction of labor is not contraindicated with a prior cesarean delivery, it makes VBAC success less likely and therefore should be considered in the counseling process. The importance of dynamic counseling cannot be underestimated. The need for induction may arise or, conversely, the patient may present in spontaneous labor and may change a physician's previous recommendations.

Number of Prior Cesareans

Whereas 2 prior cesarean deliveries were previously viewed as a contraindication to TOLAC, more recent data suggest that these patients may be candidates for a TOLAC attempt. A recent meta-analysis of patients attempting VBAC after 2 prior vaginal deliveries noted a VBAC success rate of 71.1% and a uterine rupture rate of 1.36%.[32] These results are similar to those of patients with one prior cesarean section. Other studies have reported high VBAC success rates in patients with 2 or more cesareans compared with women with only one prior cesarean section.[12,33] There are also data to suggest that patients with 3 prior cesarean deliveries have similar success rates for vaginal delivery to women with one prior cesarean delivery. In a retrospective review by Cahill and colleagues,[34] 860 women with 3 or more prior cesarean sections were evaluated. Eighty-nine of these women had a TOLAC with a success rate for VBAC of 79.8% and no cases of uterine rupture. Together, these studies continue to support the fact that the overall risk of uterine rupture is low, even in women with more than one prior cesarean, and that while remaining part of the important counseling, focus should be shifted to identifying patients who would be good candidates for VBAC success. In accordance with some of the aforementioned findings of a low risk of uterine rupture with similar rates of VBAC success, ACOG supports women with 1 or 2 prior cesareans as candidates for a TOLAC.[13]

Indication for Cesarean Section

A detailed obstetric history will help counsel women contemplating a TOLAC. It has been clearly demonstrated that the indication for previous cesarean section affects the future in VBAC success. For patients who have a nonrecurring indication, such as breech presentation or nonreassuring fetal status, chances of VBAC success are higher than with other indications that could recur such as arrest disorders and labor dystocia.[35] This approach is intuitive, as factors that contributed to the initial cesarean delivery, such as limited pelvic capacity, may still be present.

Of interest, augmentation in the index pregnancy that resulted in cesarean delivery has also been associated with a decreased VBAC success rate. Spaans and colleagues[36] evaluated the labor patterns in the index pregnancy and the rate of VBAC success in subsequent pregnancies. Two hundred and fourteen women were evaluated. Sixty-eight percent attempted a TOLAC and 71.4% were successful. Oxytocin use (OR 3.1, 95% CI 1.4–7.1), contractions longer than 12 hours (OR 3.0, 95% CI 1.3–7.0), and dilation less than 1 cm/h (OR 5.6, 95% CI 1.1–39.4) were all associated with decreased of VBAC success in future pregnancies.

Using 60% to 80% VBAC success rate as a general reference, women with a nonrecurring indication represent the upper end of this range. For recurring indications, success rates are clearly lower.

Maternal Age

In determining a patient's risk, maternal age may assist in counseling. Srinivas and colleagues[37] estimated the effect of maternal age on VBAC success. Using the age range 21 to 34 as a reference group, women aged 15 to 20 years were 27% less likely to have a failed VBAC. Compared with women younger than 35 years, women older than 35 were more likely to experience an unsuccessful trial of labor (OR 1.14, 95% CI 1.03–1.25) and were 39% more likely to experience VBAC-related complications.

Uterine Anomalies

Many women are diagnosed with a uterine anomaly at the time of their index cesarean section and request information for a subsequent pregnancy. This situation was evaluated by a retrospective, population-based study by Erez and colleagues[38] to determine the rate of success and complications in patients with Mullerian anomalies undergoing a TOLAC. There were 165 women in the cohort of 5571 eligible patients. The VBAC success rate was 37.6% for women with Mullerian anomalies and 50.7% for those with a normal uterus (P<.0009). There were 10 cases of uterine rupture; however, these all occurred in women with a normal uterus. Women with a uterine anomaly should be counseled that based on the small amount of data available on their relatively rare condition, their risk of uterine rupture is low but they may have an increased risk of failed TOLAC.

Macrosomia

The effect of fetal size was evaluated by Peaceman and colleagues[39] using the MFMU Cesarean Registry. The investigators specifically studied patients whose prior cesarean delivery was performed for dystocia, defined as a failed induction, cephalopelvic disproportion, failure to progress, or failed forceps or vacuum. VBAC success in a subsequent pregnancy was 54% if the previous cesarean was performed for dystocia. This result contrasted with 67% for other indications (P<.01). Of interest, if the fetal weight of the current pregnancy attempting VBAC exceeded the initial pregnancy by 500 g, the success rate was only 38%. The odds of success decreased 3.8% for every increase of 100 g.

Older retrospective analyses of VBAC attempts noted that infants with birth weights of more than 4000 g were less likely to deliver vaginally.[40,41] The fetal size in the current pregnancy can therefore be used to assist clinical decision making and mode of delivery.

Maternal Body Mass Index

Maternal obesity and diabetes both appear to adversely affect VBAC success rates.[42] Juhasz and colleagues[43] evaluated VBAC success rates and stratified these by body mass index (BMI; calculated as the weight in kilograms divided by height in meters squared, ie, kg/m²). A total of 1213 women were evaluated. The success rate for a BMI less than 19.8 was 83.1%. This figure decreased as BMI increased. For BMI 19.8 to 26, the success rate decreased to 79.9%. For BMI 26.1 to 29, the rate decreased further to 69.3%. For BMI greater than 29, the rate was 68.2% (P<.001).

A retrospective analysis by Durnwald and colleagues[44] also evaluated the VBAC success rate in obese and overweight women. Of 510 women in their cohort with one prior cesarean delivery who attempted a TOLAC, 337 (66%) were successful. The success rate was significantly lower for women with a BMI greater than 30 (54.6%, P = .003) compared with women with a normal BMI (70.5%). Of interest, women who gained weight between pregnancies also had a decreased VBAC success rate. Women whose BMI was normal but became overweight (BMI 25–29.9) before their second pregnancy had a 56.6% VBAC success rate. This finding was in contrast to women who remained at a normal BMI, who had a success rate of 74.2% (P = .006).

Other studies have correlated the adverse effect of maternal obesity on VBAC success. Landon and colleagues[27] evaluated multiple factors in determining VBAC success rate. The overall VBAC success rate in obese women (BMI >30) was 68.4%, compared with a rate of 79.6% in nonobese women (P<.001).

Carroll and colleagues[45] evaluated the VBAC success rate by maternal prepregnancy weight. For patients weighing less than 200 lb (91 kg), the VBAC success rate was 81.8%. The success rate was lower for women between 200 and 300 lb (91–136 kg), at 57.1%. It was lowest for women heavier than 300 lb (136 kg), at 13.3% (P = .001). Infectious morbidity was also greatest in obese women, at 39%. The infectious morbidity for lean women was 5.7% (P = .001). In another retrospective cohort study, the VBAC failure rate was higher for pregestational diabetics than for nondiabetics (38% vs 24%, P<.001).[46] Women with increased BMI clearly experience decreased VBAC success rates.

Ethnicity

Gestational diabetes and preeclampsia are just two pregnancy-related conditions that are increased in certain ethnicities.[47,48] VBAC success rates also can be added to this list. Hollard and colleagues[49] used a retrospective cohort study to determine the odds of VBAC success for multiple ethnicities. These investigators found a significant difference between Caucasians, Hispanics, and African Americans in terms of VBAC success (79.3%, 79.3%, and 70%, respectively). When compared with Caucasian women, the adjusted odds ratio for African American women was 0.37 (95% CI 0.27–0.5), and 0.63 (95% CI 0.51–0.79) for Hispanic women. Although there are likely confounders within the VBAC success rate, maternal ethnicity does seem to affect the rate of success.[50]

Prematurity

Whereas postdates has been associated with a nonstatistically significant decrease in VBAC success, prematurity has been associated with an increase in VBAC success rate. A large retrospective analysis by Quinones and colleagues[51] evaluated 20,156 women with a prior cesarean section. TOLAC was attempted in 61%. The VBAC success rate for term and preterm was 74% and 82%, respectively (P<.001). Multivariable analysis showed that the VBAC was higher in preterm gestations (adjusted OR 1.54, 95% CI 1.27–1.86).

The MFMU Network observational study evaluated the rates of VBAC success and risks associated with TOLAC for preterm pregnancies with a prior cesarean delivery.[52] A total of 2338 preterm women with a history of cesarean delivery underwent a TOLAC. The VBAC success rate was similar in a comparison of the preterm group with a term cohort of 15,331 women (72.8% vs 73.3%, $P = .64$). The rates of uterine rupture (0.34% vs 0.74%, $P = .03$) and dehiscence (0.26% vs 0.67%, $P = .02$) were lower for the preterm delivery when compared with term delivery. The patient with a prior cesarean who presents preterm should be informed that early gestational age is not a contraindication to a VBAC attempt.

Interpregnancy Interval

Previous studies have been performed to address the impact of interpregnancy interval. Huang and colleagues[53] used a large cohort of patients with one prior cesarean section to determine the influence of interpregnancy interval on VBAC success. A total of 1516 patients were evaluated with complete information for 1185. The VBAC success rate was 79.0% for patients with an interpregnancy delivery interval of less than 19 months. The success rate was not significantly different for patients with an interpregnancy interval greater than 19 months (85.5%, $P = .12$). However, women with an interpregnancy interval of less than 19 months who underwent induction had a decreased VBAC success rate compared with patients who presented in spontaneous labor. The results of this study underscore the importance of spontaneous labor in terms of VBAC success.

ALGORITHMS

Multiple investigators have attempted to create formulas to calculate individual specific results, and these have been achieved with varying degrees of success. Costantine and colleagues[54] used a cohort of term women with a history of one prior cesarean delivery to create a prediction model. Variables analyzed included age, BMI, ethnicity, prior vaginal delivery, prior VBAC, and indication for prior cesarean delivery. This model found that women's predicted rate of success did not significantly differ from their predicted rate when it was below 50%. The success rates were approximately 10% to 20% lower for women with predicted VBAC success rates of greater than 50%.

Grobman and colleagues[25] also created a nomogram using factors available at the first prenatal visit. A total of 7660 women were available in this analysis, and factors evaluated included many of the variables mentioned in this article. Maternal age, BMI, ethnicity, prior vaginal delivery, and indication were all components of the logistic regression analysis. The investigators concluded that the nomogram was accurate and discriminating, and was a potentially useful tool for patient-specific rates of success.

Other useful equations are accessible via the Internet.[25] Physicians can enter patient demographic information to obtain a "VBAC success rate" for a patient. Patients whose value is greater than 50% in achieving VBAC are deemed appropriate candidates. While this information is useful, it has yet to be validated and may not perform any better than simple clinical acumen. If a woman presents with a 60% to 80% rate of VBAC success, the clinician must identify factors that place the patient at either end of this range of predicted VBAC success.

PRACTICAL APPLICATION

The woman who presents for care with a history of cesarean delivery is common in clinical practice. Practitioners must bear in mind that a successful VBAC carries the least morbidity for the woman with a history of cesarean, and that patient selection is paramount. As important is highlighting the range of success while individualizing risk estimation for each patient. The two most dominant factors that positively influence success are at least one prior vaginal birth and spontaneous labor. A detailed history indicating the circumstances around the index delivery are crucial for assessing the patient's risk and, ultimately, the likelihood of success in achieving a VBAC. Inquiries regarding fetal status and cervical dilation at the time of cesarean are important for appropriate counseling. The goal of counseling is to not only identify women for potential TOLAC but also identify those that are unlikely to have VBAC success. Induction of labor, recurrent indication for cesarean delivery, morbid obesity, and fetal macrosomia are just some of the factors that can affect success and influence decision making.

It is also desirable to be flexible in formulating plans regarding the mode of delivery. A woman with 2 prior cesarean sections may be a poor VBAC candidate if she requires an induction of labor. However, should she present in spontaneous labor at 5-cm dilation, her risk profile and success rate change dramatically. Flexibility will allow clinicians the ability to achieve the goal of increasing the number of successful VBACs and decreasing the cesarean delivery rate.

SUMMARY

The dictum "once a cesarean, always a cesarean" still resonates despite a lack of evidence suggesting that this should be the case. It has been demonstrated that women who undergo successful VBAC have lower short-term and long-term morbidity. Conversely, women who are unsuccessful following TOLAC have the highest morbidity. Identifying the best candidates using factors available to the obstetrician can serve the dual goal of increasing the VBAC success rate while minimizing maternal morbidity.

REFERENCES

1. Centers for Disease Control and Prevention (CDC). Rates of cesarean delivery—United States, 1991. MMWR Morb Mortal Wkly Rep 1993;42(15):285–9.
2. Martin JA, Hamilton BE, Sutton PD, et al. Births: final data for 2005. Natl Vital Stat Rep 2007;56(6):1–103.
3. Gregory KD, Fridman M, Korst L. Trends and patterns of vaginal birth after cesarean availability in the United States. Semin Perinatol 2010;34(4):237–43.
4. Yeh J, Wactawski-Wende J, Shelton JA, et al. Temporal trends in the rates of trial of labor in low-risk pregnancies and their impact on the rates and success of vaginal birth after cesarean delivery. Am J Obstet Gynecol 2006;194(1):144.
5. Pare E, Quinones JN, Macones GA. Vaginal birth after caesarean section versus elective repeat caesarean section: assessment of maternal downstream health outcomes. BJOG 2006;113(1):75–85.
6. O'Brien-Abel N. Uterine rupture during VBAC trial of labor: risk factors and fetal response. J Midwifery Womens Health 2003;48(4):249–57.
7. McMahon MJ, Luther ER, Bowes WA Jr, et al. Comparison of a trial of labor with an elective second cesarean section. N Engl J Med 1996;335(10):689–95.
8. Landon MB, Hauth JC, Leveno KJ, et al. Maternal and perinatal outcomes associated with a trial of labor after prior cesarean delivery. N Engl J Med 2004; 351(25):2581–9.
9. Scott JR. Avoiding labor problems during vaginal birth after cesarean delivery. Clin Obstet Gynecol 1997;40(3):533–41.
10. Pridjian G. Labor after prior cesarean section. Clin Obstet Gynecol 1992;35(3): 445–56.

11. Landon MB, Spong CY, Thom E, et al. Risk of uterine rupture with a trial of labor in women with multiple and single prior cesarean delivery. Obstet Gynecol 2006; 108(1):12–20.
12. Macones GA, Cahill A, Pare E, et al. Obstetric outcomes in women with two prior cesarean deliveries: is vaginal birth after cesarean delivery a viable option? Am J Obstet Gynecol 2005;192(4):1223–8 [discussion: 1228–9].
13. American College of Obstetricians and Gynecologists. ACOG Practice bulletin no. 115: vaginal birth after previous cesarean delivery. Obstet Gynecol 2010; 116(2 Pt 1):450–63.
14. Ritchie EH. Pregnancy after rupture of the pregnant uterus. A report of 36 pregnancies and a study of cases reported since 1932. J Obstet Gynaecol Br Commonw 1971;78(7):642–8.
15. Reyes-Ceja L, Cabrera R, Insfran E, et al. Pregnancy following previous uterine rupture. Study of 19 patients. Obstet Gynecol 1969;34(3):387–9.
16. ACOG Committee on Obstetric Practice. ACOG Committee Opinion No. 340. Mode of term singleton breech delivery. Obstet Gynecol 2006;108(1):235–7.
17. Tripathi JB, Doshi HU, Kotdawala PJ. Vaginal birth after one caesarean section: analysis of indicators of success. J Indian Med Assoc 2006;104(3):113–5.
18. Pathadey SD, Van Woerden HC, Jenkinson SD. Induction of labour after a previous caesarean section: a retrospective study in a district general hospital. J Obstet Gynaecol 2005;25(7):662–5.
19. Holt VL, Mueller BA. Attempt and success rates for vaginal birth after caesarean section in relation to complications of the previous pregnancy. Paediatr Perinat Epidemiol 1997;11(Suppl 1):63–72.
20. Gregory KD, Korst LM, Fridman M, et al. Vaginal birth after cesarean: clinical risk factors associated with adverse outcome. Am J Obstet Gynecol 2008;198(4):452. e1–10; [discussion: 452. e10–2].
21. Weinstein D, Benshushan A, Tanos V, et al. Predictive score for vaginal birth after cesarean section. Am J Obstet Gynecol 1996;174(1 Pt 1):192–8.
22. Jakobi P, Weissman A, Peretz BA, et al. Evaluation of prognostic factors for vaginal delivery after cesarean section. J Reprod Med 1993;38(9):729–33.
23. Pickhardt MG, Martin JN Jr, Meydrech EF, et al. Vaginal birth after cesarean delivery: are there useful and valid predictors of success or failure? Am J Obstet Gynecol 1992;166(6 Pt 1):1811–5 [discussion: 1815–9].
24. Mankuta DD, Leshno MM, Menasche MM, et al. Vaginal birth after cesarean section: trial of labor or repeat cesarean section? A decision analysis. Am J Obstet Gynecol 2003;189(3):714–9.
25. Grobman WA, Lai Y, Landon MB, et al. Development of a nomogram for prediction of vaginal birth after cesarean delivery. Obstet Gynecol 2007;109(4): 806–12.
26. Mercer BM, Gilbert S, Landon MB, et al. Labor outcomes with increasing number of prior vaginal births after cesarean delivery. Obstet Gynecol 2008;111(2 Pt 1): 285–91.
27. Landon MB, Leindecker S, Spong CY, et al. The MFMU Cesarean Registry: factors affecting the success of trial of labor after previous cesarean delivery. Am J Obstet Gynecol 2005;193(3 Pt 2):1016–23.
28. Cahill AG, Stamilio DM, Odibo AO, et al. Is vaginal birth after cesarean (VBAC) or elective repeat cesarean safer in women with a prior vaginal delivery? Am J Obstet Gynecol 2006;195(4):1143–7.
29. Lydon-Rochelle MT, Cahill AG, Spong CY. Birth after previous cesarean delivery: short-term maternal outcomes. Semin Perinatol 2010;34(4):249–57.

30. Sims EJ, Newman RB, Hulsey TC. Vaginal birth after cesarean: to induce or not to induce. Am J Obstet Gynecol 2001;184(6):1122–4.
31. Rosen MG, Dickinson JC. Vaginal birth after cesarean: a meta-analysis of indicators for success. Obstet Gynecol 1990;76(5 Pt 1):865–9.
32. Tahseen S, Griffiths M. Vaginal birth after two caesarean sections (VBAC-2)—a systematic review with meta-analysis of success rate and adverse outcomes of VBAC-2 versus VBAC-1 and repeat (third) caesarean sections. BJOG 2010; 117(1):5–19.
33. Miller DA, Diaz FG, Paul RH. Vaginal birth after cesarean: a 10-year experience. Obstet Gynecol 1994;84(2):255–8.
34. Cahill AG, Tuuli M, Odibo AO, et al. Vaginal birth after caesarean for women with three or more prior cesareans: assessing safety and success. BJOG 2010; 117(4):422–7.
35. Bujold E, Gauthier RJ. Should we allow a trial of labor after a previous cesarean for dystocia in the second stage of labor? Obstet Gynecol 2001;98(4):652–5.
36. Spaans WA, Sluijs MB, van Roosmalen J, et al. Risk factors at caesarean section and failure of subsequent trial of labour. Eur J Obstet Gynecol Reprod Biol 2002; 100(2):163–6.
37. Srinivas SK, Stamilio DM, Sammel MD, et al. Vaginal birth after caesarean delivery: does maternal age affect safety and success? Paediatr Perinat Epidemiol 2007;21(2):114–20.
38. Erez O, Dukler D, Novack L, et al. Trial of labor and vaginal birth after cesarean section in patients with uterine Mullerian anomalies: a population-based study. Am J Obstet Gynecol 2007;196(6):537, e1–11.
39. Peaceman AM, Gersnoviez R, Landon MB, et al. The MFMU Cesarean Registry: impact of fetal size on trial of labor success for patients with previous cesarean for dystocia. Am J Obstet Gynecol 2006;195(4):1127–31.
40. Yetman TJ, Nolan TE. Vaginal birth after cesarean section: a reappraisal of risk. Am J Obstet Gynecol 1989;161(5):1119–23.
41. Whiteside DC, Mahan CS, Cook JC. Factors associated with successful vaginal delivery after cesarean section. J Reprod Med 1983;28(11):785–8.
42. Brill Y, Windrim R. Vaginal birth after Caesarean section: review of antenatal predictors of success. J Obstet Gynaecol Can 2003;25(4):275–86.
43. Juhasz G, Gyamfi C, Gyamfi P, et al. Effect of body mass index and excessive weight gain on success of vaginal birth after cesarean delivery. Obstet Gynecol 2005;106(4):741–6.
44. Durnwald CP, Ehrenberg HM, Mercer BM. The impact of maternal obesity and weight gain on vaginal birth after cesarean section success. Am J Obstet Gynecol 2004;191(3):954–7.
45. Carroll CS Sr, Magann EF, Chauhan SP, et al. Vaginal birth after cesarean section versus elective repeat cesarean delivery: weight-based outcomes. Am J Obstet Gynecol 2003;188(6):1516–20 [discussion: 1520–2].
46. Dharan VB, Srinivas SK, Parry S, et al. Pregestational diabetes: a risk factor for vaginal birth after cesarean section failure? Am J Perinatol 2010;27(3):265–70.
47. ACOG Committee on Practice Bulletins. ACOG practice bulletin. Clinical management guidelines for obstetrician-gynecologists. number 60, March 2005. Pregestational diabetes mellitus. Obstet Gynecol 2005;105(3):675–85.
48. ACOG Committee on Practice Bulletins. ACOG practice bulletin. Diagnosis and management of preeclampsia and eclampsia. Number 33, January 2002. American College of Obstetricians and Gynecologists. Int J Gynaecol Obstet 2002; 77(1):67–75.

49. Hollard AL, Wing DA, Chung JH, et al. Ethnic disparity in the success of vaginal birth after cesarean delivery. J Matern Fetal Neonatal Med 2006;19(8):483–7.
50. Cahill AG, Stamilio DM, Odibo AO, et al. Racial disparity in the success and complications of vaginal birth after cesarean delivery. Obstet Gynecol 2008; 111(3):654–8.
51. Quinones JN, Stamilio DM, Pare E, et al. The effect of prematurity on vaginal birth after cesarean delivery: success and maternal morbidity. Obstet Gynecol 2005; 105(3):519–24.
52. Durnwald CP, Rouse DJ, Leveno KJ, et al. The Maternal-Fetal Medicine Units Cesarean Registry: safety and efficacy of a trial of labor in preterm pregnancy after a prior cesarean delivery. Am J Obstet Gynecol 2006;195(4):1119–26.
53. Huang WH, Nakashima DK, Rumney PJ, et al. Interdelivery interval and the success of vaginal birth after cesarean delivery. Obstet Gynecol 2002;99(1): 41–4.
54. Costantine MM, Fox K, Byers BD, et al. Validation of the prediction model for success of vaginal birth after cesarean delivery. Obstet Gynecol 2009;114(5): 1029–33.
55. Grobman WA, Lai Y, Landon MB, et al. Does information available at admission for delivery improve prediction of vaginal birth after cesarean? Am J Perinatol 2009;26(10):693–701.
56. Kiran TS, Chui YK, Bethel J, et al. Is gestational age an independent variable affecting uterine scar rupture rates? Eur J Obstet Gynecol Reprod Biol 2006; 126(1):68–71.
57. Kraiem J, Ben Brahim Y, Chaabane K, et al. [Indicators for successful vaginal delivery after cesarean section: a proposal of a predictive score]. Tunis Med 2006;84(1):16–20.
58. Dodd J, Crowther C. Vaginal birth after Caesarean versus elective repeat Caesarean for women with a single prior Caesarean birth: a systematic review of the literature. Aust N Z J Obstet Gynaecol 2004;44(5):387–91.
59. Upadhyaya CD, Upadhyaya DM, Carlan SJ. Vaginal birth after cesarean delivery in a small rural community with a solo practice. Am J Perinatol 2003;20(2):63–7.
60. Nassar AH, Adra AM, Chakhtoura N, et al. Severe preeclampsia remote from term: labor induction or elective cesarean delivery? Am J Obstet Gynecol 1998;179(5):1210–3.
61. Boulvain M, Fraser WD, Brisson-Carroll G, et al. Trial of labour after caesarean section in sub-Saharan Africa: a meta-analysis. Br J Obstet Gynaecol 1997; 104(12):1385–90.
62. Bhal PS, Sharma A, Asaad K. Vaginal delivery after caesarean section: factors influencing success rates. Aust N Z J Obstet Gynaecol 1996;36(4):497–8.
63. Lovell R. Vaginal delivery after Caesarean section: factors influencing success rates. Aust N Z J Obstet Gynaecol 1996;36(1):4–8.

Can a Vaginal Birth After Cesarean Delivery be a Normal Labor and Birth? Lessons from Midwifery Applied to Trial of Labor After a Previous Cesarean Delivery

Tekoa L. King, CNM, MPH*

KEYWORDS

- Vaginal birth after cesarean • Informed consent
- Prenatal counseling • Intrapartum care

The cesarean delivery rate has dramatically increased in the United States over the last 15 years. In 1996, the overall cesarean delivery rate was 20.7%, and by 2008 it had increased 50% to a record high of 32.3% of all births.[1,2] As the number of cesarean births has increased, the adverse effects of this surgical procedure have also become apparent, which has recently reignited efforts to decrease the cesarean delivery rate.[3] Repeat cesareans account for 30.9% of the indications for cesarean delivery,[2] thus increasing the vaginal birth after cesarean delivery (VBAC) rate is one of the most important ways to reduce the overall cesarean delivery rate.

Pregnant women who had a cesarean delivery in a previous birth must choose between an elective repeat cesarean delivery (ERCD) or a trial of labor after cesarean (TOLAC). There are multiple considerations that affect this decision, including an individualized risk of uterine rupture and chance of VBAC success, access to intrapartum care if she wants a TOLAC, and her personal desires for how her labor and birth

The author has nothing to disclose.
Department of Obstetrics, Gynecology and Reproductive Medicine, University of California San Francisco, CA, USA
* 4265 Fruitvale Avenue, Oakland CA 94602.
E-mail address: tking@acnm.org

Clin Perinatol 38 (2011) 247–263
doi:10.1016/j.clp.2011.03.003
0095-5108/11/$ – see front matter © 2011 Elsevier Inc. All rights reserved.

proceed. Although there are several recent publications that summarize recommended prenatal counseling,[4] most focus primarily on the risk of uterine rupture and the chance of VBAC success.[5,6] Antepartum and intrapartum care practices that might improve maternal satisfaction and/or vaginal delivery rates have not been given much attention in the context of VBAC. This article reviews evidence-based antepartum and intrapartum care practices that are known to improve maternal satisfaction and/or vaginal birth rates and explores how these care practices can be adapted for the woman undergoing a TOLAC. Although many of these techniques are frequently identified with midwifery care practices, they are found in many settings that focus on family-centered care.

Nationally, the proportion of women who attempt TOLAC after a previous cesarean delivery is approximately 17% to 28.8%, but there is wide regional and institutional variation.[2,7] Western states have the highest VBAC rate and southern states have the lowest, with the northeast and midwest statistically between the west and south. Tertiary academic hospitals, teaching hospitals, and public hospitals have higher rates of VBAC than do community settings. DeFranco and colleagues[8] conducted a retrospective cohort study of women who were offered VBAC in 17 hospitals in Pennsylvania between 1996 and 2000 (n = 25,065) and found the VBAC attempt rate was 61% in university hospitals and 50.4% in community hospitals.

VBAC rates seem to be higher when the provider is a family physician or certified nurse-midwife rather than an obstetrician.[9,10] Although the reason for these differences is not known, survey data from the American College of Obstetricians and Gynecologists (ACOG) has found that ACOG members are performing fewer VBACs secondary to concerns about medical liability and restricted access at their delivery settings.[11] In the 2005 Listening to Mothers Survey, 57% of the women interested in VBAC were denied the option of TOLAC.[12] The top 3 reasons for the denial were: caregiver unwillingness (45%), unwillingness of hospital (23%), and medical reason (11%).

VBAC success rates are not significantly affected by regional, institutional, or provider characteristics. Approximately 60% to 80% of women who undergo TOLAC have a successful VBAC.[3] Similarly, uterine rupture, which is arguably the most morbid complication of TOLAC, has remained stable at less than 1%.[3] Thus the variability in VBAC rates seems to be primarily related to a decrease in TOLAC rather than a decrease in VBAC success.

FACTORS THAT AFFECT DECISION MAKING ABOUT TOLAC VERSUS ERCD

Given a high VBAC success rate and low complication rates, factors that affect the choice a woman makes and factors that affect her experience deserve heightened scrutiny. Approximately half of women who have had a cesarean birth make their decision about future mode of birth before becoming pregnant again, and another 34% to 39% make their decision around the midpoint of the subsequent pregnancy.[13] Women attempt to balance risks to themselves versus risks to their fetus and factor in beliefs about their previous birth experience, family influences, and societal or cultural influences, a process that can engender a high degree of decisional conflict.[14,15] Therefore, it is worth reviewing what is known in general about how pregnant women assess risk and make health decisions.

First, most pregnant women are willing to tolerate a high degree of risk to themselves in exchange for no risk for their baby.[16-18] The health risks for the mother are higher with ERCD and the health risks to the fetus are higher with TOLAC.[3] This is the primary reason why the risks associated with ERCD and the risks associated with TOLAC are not comparable for the woman who is making this decision. Although the absolute risk of uterine rupture and fetal death associated with TOLAC is numerically lower by 2 to 3 orders of magnitude than the chance of maternal morbidities associated with ERCD,[3,18] most women do not initially or instinctively balance the numeric risks. In addition, the cultural goal in the United States is a zero-risk baby, and women generally choose options that avoid any risk to the fetus without knowing or understanding the numeric values involved.

Second, once a woman makes a choice about planned or hoped-for mode of birth, that choice becomes her expectation for how she gives birth. Because personal expectations are one of the most important factors that determine patient satisfaction with care during labor and birth, the process of making this decision can have a significant effect on ultimate satisfaction with the care rendered both prenatally and during the intrapartum period.[19] In addition to these 2 generalities, several specific factors influence VBAC decision making.

The Effect of the Previous Cesarean Delivery

Every birth is a watershed event for the individual parturient. Women remember details of their labor and births for many years and seem to have the most accurate memories of cesarean deliveries.[20–22] In a unique analysis of childbirth satisfaction reported by 1451 women 2 months and then 1 year after giving birth, Waldenstrom[23] found that women who had a cesarean delivery were more likely to change their opinion from positive to negative or mixed feelings when compared with women who had a vaginal birth. In addition, the incidence of postpartum depressed mood, posttraumatic stress syndrome, and negative perceptions of birth are increased after cesarean delivery when compared with the postpartum psychosocial function in women who give birth vaginally.[24,25] This finding seems to be especially true for women who had an emergency cesarean delivery.[24,26,27] The sense of losing control and not being involved in the decision to undergo a cesarean delivery is the most frequently noted concern of women who report being traumatized by a cesarean birth.[28]

This body of literature confirms what most clinicians know: women who had an unscheduled cesarean birth frequently present in a subsequent pregnancy with vivid and intense feelings about their cesarean experience. These previous birth stories are the elephant in the room; they are exceedingly important, they have a powerful effect on decision making for subsequent births, and they are often unaddressed.[29,30]

Additional Personal Factors that Affect Choice of TOLAC Versus ERCD

Studies that have evaluated the reasons for choosing TOLAC or ERCD have identified several additional themes. Women who have had a previous vaginal birth and those who believe they are likely to have a successful VBAC are most likely to choose TOLAC. Additional determinants of a preference for TOLAC include: perception of family obligations, the need for a fast recovery, the desire to experience a natural birth, and a preference for partner involvement.[31,32]

Conversely, determinants of the preference for ERCD include: fear of a failed TOLAC, avoidance of labor pain, choice for postpartum tubal ligation, desire for ERCD over an emergency cesarean after a trial of labor, and/or the desire to choose a delivery date.[31,32] The belief that the chosen mode of birth is the safest is seen in both women who choose ERDC and women who choose TOLAC.[14]

Other personal factors that affect this decision include level of perceived personal efficacy, VBAC counseling programs, and patient involvement in decision making. Women who are not counseled prenatally are more likely to choose ERCD.[33,34] Most women want to be involved in the decision-making process but women have varied opinions about how much responsibility they want for the decision.[29]

Regardless of how much responsibility women want, all women studied prefer information that addresses their individual situation, which means an individualized risk assessment, and a shared decision-making process that addresses personal values and beliefs that best meet their needs.[32]

The Role of the Health Care Provider

The health care provider's recommendation is frequently cited as an important contributor to the decision about TOLAC versus ERCD, yet little is known about provider preferences for TOLAC versus VBAC.[32] However, there has been much study on communication techniques that optimize patient understanding. Accurate and objective communication of risks and benefits is dependent on (1) presentation of the information in a way the patient can perceive and understand and (2) avoidance of framing.

COMMUNICATING RISKS AND BENEFITS: HEALTH LITERACY

Antenatal counseling about TOLAC and ERCD should be evidence based and patient centered, with the goal of shared decision making.[17,32,35] There has been much research on factors that affect satisfaction with childbirth in general. Personal expectations, caregiver support, quality of caregiver support, and shared decision making consistently rate as the most important determinants of satisfaction with childbirth.[19] Each of these factors can be addressed over the course of prenatal care by listening carefully to the story of the previous cesarean and engaging in shared decision making when planning care practices that are offered during the upcoming labor. Survey and qualitative studies specific to VBAC decision making have found that women are more satisfied with their experience regardless of the type of birth they have, when they believe they were involved in the decision to the degree that was comfortable for them.[29,33]

Shared Decision Making

Shared decision making is different from presenting risks and benefits. Shared decision making is "decisions that are shared by doctor and patient and informed by best evidence, not only about risks and benefits but also patient specific characteristics and values."[36] This type of patient-centered decision making can occur when clear communication of risk, benefits, and the range of available options is presented. The decision is then made within the context of the woman's personal values, beliefs, and preferences.

Health Literacy and Health Numeracy

Accurate perception of risks and benefits of TOLAC and ERCD depends on health literacy. Health literacy is defined by the US Department of Health and Human Services as "The degree to which individuals have the capacity to obtain, process, and understand basic health information and services needed to make appropriate health decisions."[37] Approximately one-half of the adult population in the United States have low health literacy.[38] Although low health literacy is more likely in certain populations such as elderly people, and those with lower educational attainment, the use of educational attainment as a proxy for health literacy is misleading. Many persons read and comprehend below their educational level.[39]

A key component of health literacy is health numeracy, which is the degree to which individuals understand quantitative and probabilistic health information.[40] The counseling about TOLAC versus ERCD involves citing multiple statistics including the risk of uterine rupture, risk of fetal death in the event of uterine rupture, chance of VBAC success, incidence of neonatal morbidity after ERCD, the incidence of placenta previa or accreta in subsequent pregnancies, and the effect of multiple cesareans on future fertility. These numbers involve basic analytical and statistical health numeracy that requires cognition several steps beyond the usual dichotomization of risks into binary categories of high risk and low risk.[16,40] Health literacy and health numeracy can be assessed. A thorough description of the assessment tools available is beyond the scope of this article, and the interested reader is referred to recent publications by Powers and colleagues[39] and Lipkus.[41]

There are several simple techniques for communicating risk that ensure an objective approach and increase patient comprehension. Providers engaged in TOLAC versus ERCD counseling will find these tools helpful:

- Consistent use of absolute numbers in place of percentages, relative risks (RRs), or risk ratios improves accurate perception.[42]
- Avoid use of words such as "rare," "unlikely," "uncommon," or "unusual"; these are inexact concepts because 1 individual's interpretation can be different from another individual's interpretation of the same word.[43]
- It is easier to understand smaller denominators and whole numbers. For example, "2 in 100" is more accurately interpreted than "18 to 20 in 1000." Use the same numeric denominator whenever possible.
- Round numbers and avoid the use of decimals.[41]
- The use of visual tools such as the Paling Perspective Scale[44] or others like it help the patient see both the chance that an adverse outcome will occur and the chance that an adverse outcome will not occur. Using these simple techniques helps improve risk communication for most individuals regardless of attained educational level. These tools help the provider avoid framing.

Framing

Framing is defined as "the presentation of two logically equivalent situations, where one is presented in positive or gain terms and the other in negative or loss terms."[45] Gain frames (probability of success) tend to engender greater compliance than loss frames (probability of failure). In the case of VBAC decision making, saying that 7 of 10 women have a successful VBAC is the same as saying there is a 30% chance of failure. However, the first format makes the chance of success seem higher to most audiences. Individuals who have low educational attainment and those who have low health numeracy are more vulnerable to framing effects when compared with individuals with higher levels of education and a better ability to interpret numbers.[46,47] One well-documented way to decrease the effects of framing in addition to the use of absolute numbers and natural frequencies is the use of visual decision aids.

Decision Aids

Decision aids are brochures, videos, or computer programs that help individuals make a decision about medical options wherein there is no clear advantage to one or the other choice, both have benefits and harms, and in situations in which individuals have differing preferences and values that affect their rating of the option. The use of decision aids to assist persons making complex health decisions is a young science that is receiving research attention and has been the subject of 1 Cochrane review.[48] Decision aids in general improve knowledge and accurate understanding of risk. In addition, they reduce decisional conflict and increase perceived participation in decision making.[48]

Several studies have evaluated the efficacy of different decision aids for women choosing TOLAC or ERCD.[14,18,44,49–51] Shorten and colleagues[51] conducted a randomized controlled trial (n = 227) that evaluated the effect of a decision-aid booklet, which described the risks and benefits of TOLAC and ERCD and included some value clarification exercises. The group that read the decision-aid booklet had improved knowledge scores (2.17 vs 42, respectively, difference in mean increase was 1.75, 95% confidence interval [CI] 1.15–2.35, P<.001) and decreased decisional conflict (−0,40 vs −0.08, respectively, 95% CI for intervention group change in score −0.51 to −0.29, P<.001). However, it was not clear if this booklet had any effect on the decision that was made.

More complex computer decision-analysis aids have also been evaluated for the TOLAC versus ERCD choice.[50,52] All seem to reduce decisional conflict and improve knowledge. Those decision aids that present risk as a numeric scale (the operator can choose any point along a scale from "extremely important to avoid side effect" to "extremely important to have a good delivery experience") seem to be more reliable than those that use a discrete text-anchored format (the operator can choose discrete text phrases to signify preferences such as "extremely important," "equally important," "much more important").[52] A randomized controlled trial by Montgomery and colleagues[50] found the decision aid that helped prioritize preferences about health outcomes had a larger effect on the decision about mode of birth when compared with the decision aid that presented risk probabilities.

More recently Sharma and colleagues[18] compared 2 computer decision aids. One generated a recommended mode of birth derived from the participant's priority for avoiding maternal and fetal risks and priorities for the birth experience. The second decision aid generated a recommended mode of birth that was derived from a decision tree based on absolute risks that then had individual priorities factored in. The first decision aid resulted in a recommendation for ERCD for 73% of the participants and the second resulted in a recommendation for TOLAC for 82% of the participants. The investigators found that the first decision aid led to more recommendations for ERCD because women prioritized avoiding death/disability for the infant over all other criteria. In contrast the second decision aid favored TOLAC because the absolute risk values favor TOLAC over ERCD with regard to fewer health risks. Although decision aids clearly improve knowledge and reduce decisional conflict, there are substantive differences in how they affect the choice about mode of birth; the decision aids that are more complex than the Paling Perspective Scale may not be ready for widespread clinical implementation.

CONTENT OF ANTEPARTUM COUNSELING ABOUT TOLAC VERSUS ERCD

Traditionally the decision about TOLAC versus ERCD is made after the clinician determines there are no contraindications and shares the risks of TOLAC and the likelihood of successful VBAC. The classic and uncontested medical and obstetric contraindications for TOLAC are previous uterine rupture, previous classic incision or T incision, or extensive transfundal uterine surgery, medical, or obstetric complications that preclude vaginal birth.[35] Many of the factors that affect the likelihood of success and risk of uterine rupture have been identified and are reviewed elsewhere.[3–5] **Table 1** summarizes the relevant statistics associated with important maternal and newborn outcomes of TOLAC and ERCD. The quality of evidence for each of these outcomes was assessed by the 2010 National Institutes of Health Consensus Development Conference on Vaginal Birth after Cesarean.[3] Although some topics have a low level of quality in that there were no randomized controlled trials that

Table 1 Risks associated with TOLAC and ERCD		
Outcome	TOLAC	ERCD
Chance of VBAC success	70%	N/A
Short-term effects: maternal		
Risk of uterine rupture	3.8 per 1000 women	2.6 per 10,000 women
Maternal mortality	1.9 per 100,000 women at term	9.6 per 100,000 women at term
Hysterectomy	1.57 per 1000 women	2.8 per 1000 women
Blood transfusion	6.6 per 1000 women at term	4.6 per 1000 women at term
Operative injury	4.0–5.1 per 1000 women	2.5–4.4 per 1000 women
Infection	46 per 1000 women	32 per 1000 women
Hospital stay	2.5 days	3.92 days
Long-term effects: maternal		
Placenta previa in subsequent pregnancy	9 per 1000 women for 1 previous CD 17 per 1000 women for 2 previous CD 30 per 1000 women for 3 previous CD	
Placenta accreta	3.1 per 1000 women for 1 previous CD 5.7 per 1000 women for 2 previous CD 24 per 1000 women for ≥3 previous CD	
Urinary incontinence	No data	No data
Pelvic floor disorders	No data	No data
Short-term and long-term effects: infant		
Neonatal death rate	11 per 1000	5 per 1000
Intrapartum fetal death	20 per 100,000	zero
Hypoxic ischemic encephalopathy	46 per 100,000	zero
Respiratory problem first days after birth	Infants born by ERCD have higher rates of transient tachypnea of the newborn, respiratory distress syndrome, and need for oxygen and ventilator support when compared with newborns born after VBAC	

Abbreviations: CD, cesarean delivery; N/A, not applicable.
Data from Refs.[3,5,6,60]

documented the numeric risk, they are important to women and therefore the data that are available should be shared despite the lack of high-quality evidence.

There is a specific issue of import with regard to VBAC statistics. Many of the VBAC studies compare successful VBAC with ERCD but this is not the comparison of import for a woman who is counseled prenatally and who does not yet know how she will give birth.[3,35,53] The most adverse health outcomes occur when a woman has labor then a repeat cesarean.[54] Therefore, the data women need prenatally should come from studies that prospectively compare TOLAC with ERCD so that the statistics from women who have a failed TOLAC are captured and represented appropriately.

For the woman who has had 1 prior low transverse cesarean delivery, the risk of uterine rupture is no different than the risk of other equivalent serious adverse outcomes faced by all nulliparous women when they enter labor.[53] The overall risk of uterine rupture is 3.2/1000 women who undergo TOLAC and the risk of placental abruption is 1/100 pregnancies.[55] Likewise, the 70% chance of having a successful vaginal birth is similar to the chance that a nulliparous woman in labor at term has a vaginal birth with today's current cesarean delivery rates (76.5%).[1]

ANTENATAL COUNSELING FOR WOMEN WHO CHOOSE TOLAC

Despite risk equivalency relative to all nulliparous women, individuals who choose TOLAC must first determine if there is a setting in their geographic area where TOLAC is offered. Once a place of birth has been chosen, information about institutional procedures and the management of labor is needed.

Place of Birth for TOLAC

One example of regionalization and response to restrictive hospital policies is the Northern New England Perinatal Quality Improvement Network (NNEPQIN) (http://www.nnepqin.org/). This collaboration between hospitals in New Hampshire and Vermont reviewed the literature and developed guidelines for offering TOLAC. Women who have had a previous cesarean delivery are assigned 1 of 3 risk categories based on the number of previous cesareans, need for induction of labor, and additional obstetric or medical complications. Recommendations for the presence of obstetric and anesthesia services are made for each of the 3 risk categories. With this guideline in place, hospitals in this geographic area resumed TOLAC services for women in the lowest risk category (1 previous cesarean, spontaneous labor, no fetal heart rate abnormalities, no need for augmentation) and established a referral system to the tertiary care settings for women who were at medium or high risk. The NNEPQUIN collaboration provides a consent form and patient education form for women choosing TOLAC.

Two studies have evaluated the outcomes of women who underwent TOLAC in an out-of-hospital birthing center. Lieberman and colleagues[9] evaluated the outcomes of 1453 women who had a previous cesarean delivery and who started labor in 1 of 27 North American out-of-hospital birthing centers between 1990 and 2000. David and colleagues[56] evaluated the outcomes of 364 women who had a TOLAC in one of several out-of-hospital birthing centers in Germany between 2000 and 2004. The success and complication rates from these 2 studies are presented in **Table 2**. The overall VBAC success rate in the Lieberman study was 87%, which is higher than the success rate of 60% to 80% that has been seen in most North American studies, and the successful VBAC rate in the German study was 73.5%.[3,9,56] There were no uterine ruptures or perinatal deaths in the German study. There were 6 uterine ruptures and 7 perinatal deaths in the North American study, a uterine rupture rate of 4/1000 births, and a perinatal death rate of 5/1000 births. The investigators of the North American study recommended that women who want to have a TOLAC should not labor in out-of-hospital birthing centers. However, a detailed look at the studies suggests that their conclusion was premature.[57,58]

There were 99 women in the North American study who had more than 1 previous cesarean delivery. These women were excluded from giving birth in the birthing centers in the German study. Three of the 6 uterine ruptures in the North American study occurred in women who had more than 1 previous cesarean delivery. Of the 7 perinatal deaths that were documented in the North American study, 4 occurred in women who had 2 previous cesarean deliveries or in women who were at more than 42 weeks' gestation. If women with more than 1 previous cesarean delivery and those who were postdates were removed from the analysis, the uterine rupture rate would be 2/1000 births and the perinatal death rate would be 2/1000 births. These rates are lower than national rates for all women in comparable categories.[3,59]

The adverse outcome of import for women undergoing TOLAC is uterine rupture yet the risk that the uterus ruptures in women undergoing TOLAC is not higher than the risk of other rare obstetric emergencies (eg, placental abruption) in all other

Table 2 Studies of TOLAC in out-of-hospital settings		
Variable	Lieberman et al (n = 1453) n (%)	David et al (n = 364) n (%)
Maternal transfer to hospital during labor	347 (24)	150 (41.2)
Maternal transfer to hospital post partum	42 (4)	15 (4.1)
Emergency transfer to hospital	37 (11)	10 (2.7)
Mode of delivery		
Cesarean delivery	189 (13)	80 (22.3)
Vaginal birth in birth center	1106 (76)	214 (58.8)
Vaginal birth in hospital	158 (11)	70 (19.2)
Uterine rupture	6 (0.4)	0
Uterine rupture 1 previous cesarean (n = 1354)	3 (0.2)	0
Uterine rupture >1 previous cesarean (n = 99)	3 (3)	N/A
Maternal mortality	0	0
Perinatal mortality	7 (0.5)	0
Perinatal mortality 1 previous cesarean (n = 1354)	5 (0.3)	0
Perinatal mortality >1 previous cesarean (n = 99)	2 (2)	N/A
Perinatal mortality secondary to uterine rupture, % of all uterine ruptures	2 (28)	0

Abbreviation: N/A, not applicable.
Data from Refs.[9,25]

parturients.[3] In addition, there is no statistically significant increased risk for intrapartum perinatal death when women choosing TOLAC are compared with nulliparous women in labor.[60] Women who give birth in out-of-hospital birthing centers are not restricted to bed, they do not use epidural analgesia, they are not offered oxytocin for induction or augmentation and they are given one-to-one supportive care throughout labor. These women are usually highly screened and at low risk for maternal complications and for developing fetal acidemia during labor. Given the favorable statistics in these studies when women who are in medium-risk or higher-risk categories are not included, from these epidemiologic data, it could be argued that out-of-hospital birthing centers are better settings than hospitals for women undergoing TOLAC.

LABOR MANAGEMENT PRACTICES THAT PROMOTE VAGINAL BIRTH

Sudden fetal heart rate bradycardia is the most frequent sign of acute uterine rupture during labor.[61] For this reason, most hospitals require intravenous access (eg, heparin lock) and continuous fetal monitoring for women who are undergoing TOLAC.[62,63] Some also require an intrauterine pressure catheter in the hope of detecting sudden loss of pressure if a uterine rupture occurs. Two studies have evaluated intrauterine catheter readings before and after a uterine incision for cesarean birth[64] and before and after uterine rupture.[65] Neither found that these catheters detected loss of uterine pressure or uterine rupture. Although there is little intervention involved with having intravenous access placed, continuous electronic fetal monitoring usually requires bed rest, which disallows several labor support measures that have been documented to increase patient satisfaction and facilitate vaginal birth.

Selected evidence-based labor management practices that increase the chance of vaginal birth and those that increase the risk of cesarean delivery are listed in **Tables 3** and **4**.[9,19,56,66-77] Because the issues surrounding induction, labor progression, and monitoring are covered elsewhere in this issue, this section summarizes labor practices that reduce operative delivery rates and therefore could improve vaginal delivery rates for women undergoing TOLAC.

Active Management of Labor

The package of care practices that make up active management of labor (AML) deserves special mention. The original components of AML included: (1) one-to-one support in labor, (2) routine amniotomy, (3) oxytocin augmentation, (4) strict criteria for the diagnosis of labor, (5) strict monitoring progress in labor with use of a partogram, and (6) peer review of assisted deliveries. As a package of care, AML reduces the cesarean delivery rate (RR 0.77, 95% CI 0.63–0.94)[66] but it is a complicated

Table 3
Labor practices that promote vaginal birth

Management Practice	Comment
Active management of labor	Active management of labor modestly reduces the cesarean delivery rate but relies on a high-dose oxytocin augmentation protocol that is not recommended for women undergoing TOLAC[66]
Admit in active labor	Retrospective studies found delaying admission until active labor is established results in less intervention and lower cesarean deliveries. One randomized controlled trial of 209 women found a trend for fewer cesareans (7.6% in delayed admission group vs 10.6% in early admission group, odds ratio 0.70, 95% CI 0.27–0.81)[74]
Continuous labor support	Continuous support provided by a nonmedical person increases labor satisfaction, shortens labor length, and increases vaginal delivery rate[19]
Use of nonpharmacologic methods of pain control	Several thorough systematic reviews of various nonpharmacologic methods of pain control have been conducted.[69-71] Immersion in water, acupuncture, birthing balls, massage, and so forth are less effective pain relievers than epidural analgesia but they are associated with a high degree of patient satisfaction
Freedom of movement	Thus although studies of upright positions have not been methodologically sound enough to assess the effect on cesarean delivery, upright positions and freedom of movement are associated with less perceived pain, shorter labor, improved uterine contractility and increased patient satisfaction[68]
Delayed pushing	A meta-analysis of delayed pushing until the vertex is visible or the woman has an urge to push for women using epidural analgesia (n = 2827) found that delayed pushing increases the vaginal delivery rate (RR 1.08, 95% CI 1.01–1.15) and decreases the instrumental delivery rate (0.77, 95% CI 0.77–0.85).[77] Although there is no difference in cesarean delivery rates, avoiding an instrumental delivery is a goal of import for women undergoing TOLAC

Table 4	
Labor practices that increase the risk of cesarean delivery	
Management Practice	**Comment**
Induction of labor	Systematic analysis of expectant versus induction for women with suspected macrosomia who did not have diabetes. Expectant management associated with fewer cesarean deliveries[75]
Continuous electronic fetal monitoring (EFM)	In unselected populations, EFM is associated with an increase in cesarean delivery and no reduction in adverse neonatal outcomes.[72] There is evidence that the uterine rupture rate in carefully selected women who undergo TOLAC in settings that do not use EFM is not higher than it is in settings that do use EFM.[9,56] The optimum timing and protocol for monitoring the fetus during TOLAC have not been determined
Routine amniotomy	Although not statistically significant in a meta-analysis, there is a trend that routine amniotomy shortens labor but increases the cesarean delivery rate (n = 4893, RR 1.26, 95% CI 0.98–1.62)[73]

package of interventions that are invasive and difficult to replicate.[78] Studies and systematic reviews of individual components of AML have been conducted to determine if any one or a combination of these interventions is responsible for the noted reduction. For example, one-to-one continuous labor support is effective in reducing cesarean deliveries (n = 13,391; RR 0.91, 95% CI 0.83–0.99),[19] yet neither use of oxytocin nor amniotomy alone is effective.[79,80]

The components of AML that can facilitate vaginal birth in women undergoing TOLAC include one-to-one continuous labor support, admission when active labor has commenced,[81,82] and use of audits or peer review of operative births.[83] Conversely, the component of AML that may increase the cesarean delivery rate in women undergoing TOLAC is aggressive use of oxytocin. High-dose oxytocin protocols and maximum doses of oxytocin more than 20 mU/min seem to increase the risk of uterine rupture 4-fold (hazard ratio [HR] 3.92, 95% CI 1.06–14.52 for oxytocin dose of 21–30 mU/min and HR 4.57, 95% CI 1.00–2.82 for oxytocin dose of 31–40 mU/min).[84]

It is not clear if use of a partogram is likely to be helpful or harmful. The Friedman curve, which is the basis of most partograms, uses a cervical dilation rate of 1 cm/h, which was the slowest and still normal rate of dilation in the active phase of labor in Friedman's original studies.[85] More recent studies of nulliparous women in labor have found that the slowest and still normal rate of dilation in active labor is 0.5 cm/h.[86] Thus use of the Friedman curve to diagnose active phase arrest could increase the cesarean delivery rate for women who are in normal labor.[2] Conversely, Khan and Rizvi[87] evaluated the use of a partogram for women undergoing TOLAC (n = 236) in Karachi, Pakistan between 1988 and 1991. The alert line was 1 cm/h and the uterine rupture rate was calculated for each hour of continued labor after the alert line. There were 7 uterine ruptures (2.9%), all of which occurred between 2 and 6 hours after dilation stopped progressing. If cesarean deliveries had occurred at 2 or 3 hours after the alert line were crossed rather than later, which would have been similar to when a cesarean delivery is performed using the Friedman curve, the uterine rupture rates would have been 0.8% and 1.6%, respectively. Thus in this population, the 1 cm/h for normal progress that is used in the Friedman curve would have been protective in decreasing the uterine rupture rate.[87] Conclusions cannot be drawn from this 1 small study.

Assessing labor progress via use of a partogram was not shown to be effective in reducing the cesarean delivery rate in a Cochrane review of 5 randomized trials of women who had not had a previous cesarean delivery,[88] but because the appropriate time intervals for alert and action lines have not been determined in cohorts of women with a previous cesarean delivery or in cohorts of women without a previous cesarean delivery, more work is needed before use of partograms can be tested to determine effectiveness in preventing uterine rupture.

Midwife-led Care

Many retrospective analyses have found lower cesarean delivery rates in women cared for by midwives when compared with similar populations of women cared for by physicians in the United States.[83,89,90] A recent Cochrane review of 11 randomized trials of midwife-led care (n = 12,276) versus medical management found higher spontaneous vaginal birth rates in the group cared for by midwives (RR 1.04, 95% CI 1.02–1.06) but no statistically significant difference in cesarean delivery rates (RR 0.96, 95% CI 0.87–1.06).[91] Thus the difference was in more frequent use of instrumental deliveries by medical providers. The women cared for by midwives were more likely to feel in control during childbirth when compared with the same ratings by the women cared for by medical practitioners (RR 1.74, 95% CI 1.32–2.30). The studies that comprised this meta-analysis were from Australia and the United Kingdom, and several different midwifery models of care were included.

Midwifery care of women undergoing TOLAC comes from retrospective studies of large caseloads. In addition to the studies by Lieberman and colleagues[9] and David and colleagues[56] described earlier in this article, 1 retrospective review of women undergoing TOLAC who are cared for by midwives in the United States found a VBAC success rate of 72% (n = 649) and no uterine ruptures.[62] The data for this study were contributed by 8 different midwifery practices that were predominately hospital based, and specific care practices were not documented. Harrington and colleagues[92] reported the results of 303 women who underwent TOLAC in a hospital-based birthing center. In this practice, the policy was intermittent fetal heart rate monitoring after an initial admission evaluation with electronic fetal monitoring. All women were in spontaneous labor and admitted after active labor was established. Women with more than 1 previous low transverse scar or other medical or obstetric complication were excluded. The intrapartum transfer rate to medical management was 8.7%, which was similar to the transfer rate of women laboring in this setting who did not have a previous cesarean delivery (10.4%). VBAC occurred in 98.3% of the women undergoing TOLAC but 84% of these study patients had a previous vaginal birth in addition to a previous cesarean delivery, so a high success rate is not unexpected. There were no uterine ruptures in the women who delivered by VBAC. One asymptomatic uterine rupture was noted in 1 woman who transferred to medical management and needed oxytocin augmentation before having a repeat cesarean delivery for failure to progress. Midwifery care of women undergoing TOLAC is safe and associated with similar success rates. The uterine rupture rate in all studies conducted to date is similar to the baseline rate of less than 1% but none of the studies was big enough individually to accurately determine the incidence of this rare outcome.

The specifics of midwifery care that increases patient satisfaction and facilitates vaginal birth have not been studied. However, the midwifery model of care includes continuity of care, patient-centered care, individualized education and counseling, and minimizing unnecessary intervention that occurs within a system that supports consultation and transfer of care to medical management as needed.[93] This model is a unique fit for the needs of women undergoing TOLAC.

SUMMARY

Women who had a cesarean birth in a previous pregnancy need careful and articulate counseling prenatally to aid them in deciding about mode of delivery. If there are no contraindications to TOLAC, individuals who choose this option need access to settings that provide TOLAC. Many of these women enter labor anxious to avoid a repeat cesarean delivery. Therefore all labor support activities that support vaginal birth and/or patient satisfaction are important tools for the caregivers providing support for this population of women. The midwifery model of care incorporates many of the specific care practices that are helpful for women undergoing TOLAC. Studies of packages of care that increase vaginal birth and patient satisfaction need to be conducted.

REFERENCES

1. Martin JA, Hamilton BE, Sutton PD, et al. Births: final data for 2008. Natl Vital Stat Rep 2010;59:1–49.
2. Zhang J, Troendle J, Reddy UM, et al. Contemporary cesarean delivery practice in the United States. Am J Obstet Gynecol 2010;203(4):326.e1–10.
3. Cunningham FG, Bangdiwala S, Brown SS, et al. National Institutes of Health Consensus Development Conference Statement: vaginal birth after cesarean: new insights. March 8–10, 2010. Obstetrics & Gynecology 2010;115(6):1279–95.
4. Caughey AB. Informed consent for a vaginal birth after previous cesarean delivery. J Midwifery Womens Health 2009;54(3):249–53.
5. Guise JM, Denman MA, Emeis C, et al. Vaginal birth after cesarean: new insights on maternal and neonatal outcomes. Obstet Gynecol 2010;115(6):1267–78.
6. Landon MB. Vaginal birth after cesarean delivery. Clin Perinatol 2008;35(3): 491–504, ix–x.
7. Gregory KD, Fridman M, Korst L. Trends and patterns of vaginal birth after cesarean availability in the United States. Semin Perinatol 2010;34(4): 237–43.
8. DeFranco EA, Rampersad R, Atkins KL, et al. Do vaginal birth after cesarean outcomes differ based on hospital setting? Am J Obstet Gynecol 2007;197(4): 400.e1–6.
9. Lieberman E, Ernst EK, Rooks JP, et al. Results of the national study of vaginal birth after cesarean in birth centers. Obstet Gynecol 2004;104(5 Pt 1):933–42.
10. Russillo B, Sewitch MJ, Cardinal L, et al. Comparing rates of trial of labour attempts, VBAC success, and fetal and maternal complications among family physicians and obstetricians. J Obstet Gynaecol Can 2008;30(2):123–8.
11. Klagholz J, Strunk AL. Overview of the 2009 ACOG survey on professional liability. ACOG Clin Rev 2009;14:1–2.
12. Declercq ER, Sakala C, Corry MP, et al. Listening to mothers II. New York: Childbirth Connection; 2006.
13. Guise JM, Eden K, Emeis C, et al. Vaginal birth after cesarean: new insights. Evid Rep Technol Assess (Full Rep) 2010;191:1–397.
14. Eden KB, Hashima JN, Osterweil P, et al. Childbirth preferences after cesarean birth: a review of the evidence. Birth 2004;31(1):49–60.
15. Farnworth A, Robson SC, Thomson RG, et al. Decision support for women choosing mode of delivery after a previous caesarean section: a developmental study. Patient Educ Couns 2008;71(1):116–24.
16. Lyerly AD, Mitchell LM, Armstrong EM, et al. Risk and the pregnant body. Hastings Cent Rep 2009;39(6):34–42.

17. Lyerly AD, Mitchell LM, Armstrong EM, et al. Risks, values, and decision making surrounding pregnancy. Obstet Gynecol 2007;109(4):979–84.

18. Sharma PS, Eden KB, Guise JM, et al. Subjective risk vs. objective risk can lead to different post-cesarean birth decisions based on multiattribute modeling. J Clin Epidemiol 2011;64(1):67–78.

19. Hodnett ED, Gates S, Hofmeyr GJ, et al. Continuous support for women during childbirth. Cochrane Database Syst Rev 2007;3:CD003766.

20. Simkin P. Just another day in a woman's life? Part II: nature and consistency of women's long-term memories of their first birth experiences. Birth 1992;19(2):64–81.

21. Rice F, Lewis A, Harold G, et al. Agreement between maternal report and antenatal records for a range of pre and peri-natal factors: the influence of maternal and child characteristics. Early Hum Dev 2007;83(8):497–504.

22. Yawn BP, Suman VJ, Jacobsen SJ. Maternal recall of distant pregnancy events. J Clin Epidemiol 1998;51(5):399–405.

23. Waldenstrom U. Why do some women change their opinion about childbirth over time? Birth 2004;31(2):102–7.

24. Lobel M, DeLuca RS. Psychosocial sequelae of cesarean delivery: review and analysis of their causes and implications. Soc Sci Med 2007;64(11):2272–84.

25. Redshaw M, Hockley C. Institutional processes and individual responses: women's experiences of care in relation to cesarean birth. Birth 2010;37(2):150–9.

26. Blom EA, Jansen PW, Verhulst FC, et al. Perinatal complications increase the risk of postpartum depression. The Generation R Study. BJOG 2010;117(11):1390–8.

27. Borders N. After the afterbirth: a critical review of postpartum health relative to method of delivery. J Midwifery Womens Health 2006;51(4):242–8.

28. Porter M, van Teijlingen E, Chi Ying Yip L, et al. Satisfaction with cesarean section: qualitative analysis of open-ended questions in a large postal survey. Birth 2007;34(2):148–54.

29. Moffat MA, Bell JS, Porter MA, et al. Decision making about mode of delivery among pregnant women who have previously had a caesarean section: a qualitative study. BJOG 2007;114(1):86–93.

30. David S, Fenwick J, Bayes S, et al. A qualitative analysis of the content of telephone calls made by women to a dedicated 'Next Birth After Caesarean' antenatal clinic. Women Birth 2010;23(4):166–71.

31. Emmett CL, Shaw AR, Montgomery AA, et al. Women's experience of decision making about mode of delivery after a previous caesarean section: the role of health professionals and information about health risks. BJOG 2006;113(12):1438–45.

32. Kaimal AJ, Kuppermann M. Understanding risk, patient and provider preferences, and obstetrical decision making: approach to delivery after cesarean. Semin Perinatol 2010;34(5):331–6.

33. Cleary-Goldman J, Cornelisse K, Simpson LL, et al. Previous cesarean delivery: understanding and satisfaction with mode of delivery in a subsequent pregnancy in patients participating in a formal vaginal birth after cesarean counseling program. Am J Perinatol 2005;22(4):217–21.

34. Ridley RT, Davis PA, Bright JH, et al. What influences a woman to choose vaginal birth after cesarean? J Obstet Gynecol Neonatal Nurs 2002;31(6):665–72.

35. American College of Obstetricians and Gynecologists. ACOG practice bulletin no. 115: vaginal birth after previous cesarean delivery. Obstet Gynecol 2010;116(2 Pt 1):450–63.

36. Towle A, Godolphin W. Framework for teaching and learning informed shared decision making. BMJ 1999;319(7212):766–71.
37. US Department of Health and Human Services. Healthy people 2010: understanding and improving health. 2nd edition. Washington, DC: US Government Printing Office; 2000.
38. Nelson W, Reyna VF, Fagerlin A, et al. Clinical implications of numeracy: theory and practice. Ann Behav Med 2008;35(3):261–74.
39. Powers BJ, Trinh JV, Bosworth HB. Can this patient read and understand written health information? JAMA 2010;304(1):76–84.
40. Golbeck AL, Ahlers-Schmidt CR, Paschal AM, et al. A definition and operational framework for health numeracy. Am J Prev Med 2005;29(4):375–6.
41. Lipkus IM. Numeric, verbal, and visual formats of conveying health risks: suggested best practices and future recommendations. Med Decis Making 2007; 27(5):696–713.
42. Galesic M, Gigerenzer G, Straubinger N. Natural frequencies help older adults and people with low numeracy to evaluate medical screening tests. Med Decis Making 2009;29(3):368–71.
43. Edwards A, Elwyn G, Mulley A. Explaining risks: turning numerical data into meaningful pictures. BMJ 2002;324(7341):827–30.
44. Stallings SP, Paling JE. New tool for presenting risk in obstetrics and gynecology. Obstet Gynecol 2001;98(2):345–9.
45. Garcia-Retamero R, Galesic M. How to reduce the effect of framing on messages about health. J Gen Intern Med 2010;25(12):1323–9.
46. Garcia-Retamero R, Galesic M. Communicating treatment risk reduction to people with low numeracy skills: a cross-cultural comparison. Am J Public Health 2009;99(12):2196–202.
47. Peters E, Hart PS, Fraenkel L. Informing patients: the influence of numeracy, framing, and format of side effect information on risk perceptions. Med Decis Making 2010. [Epub ahead of print].
48. O'Connor AM, Bennett CL, Stacey D, et al. Decision aids for people facing health treatment or screening decisions. Cochrane Database Syst Rev 2009;3: CD001431.
49. Frost J, Shaw A, Montgomery A, et al. Women's views on the use of decision aids for decision making about the method of delivery following a previous caesarean section: qualitative interview study. BJOG 2009;116(7):896–905.
50. Montgomery AA, Emmett CL, Fahey T, et al. Two decision aids for mode of delivery among women with previous caesarean section: randomised controlled trial. BMJ 2007;334(7607):1305.
51. Shorten A, Shorten B, Keogh J, et al. Making choices for childbirth: a randomized controlled trial of a decision-aid for informed birth after cesarean. Birth 2005; 32(4):252–61.
52. Eden KB, Dolan JG, Perrin NA, et al. Patients were more consistent in randomized trial at prioritizing childbirth preferences using graphic-numeric than verbal formats. J Clin Epidemiol 2009;62(4):415–24, e3.
53. Rozen G, Ugoni AM, Sheehan PM. A new perspective on VBAC: a retrospective cohort study. Women Birth 2011;24(1):3–9.
54. El-Sayed YY, Watkins MM, Fix M, et al. Perinatal outcomes after successful and failed trials of labor after cesarean delivery. Am J Obstet Gynecol 2007;196(6): 583, e1–5 [discussion: 583, e5].
55. Oyelese Y, Ananth CV. Placental abruption. Obstet Gynecol 2006;108(4): 1005–16.

56. David M, Gross MM, Wiemer A, et al. Prior cesarean section–an acceptable risk for vaginal delivery at free-standing midwife-led birth centers? Results of the analysis of vaginal birth after cesarean section (VBAC) in German birth centers. Eur J Obstet Gynecol Reprod Biol 2009;142(2):106–10.

57. Albers LL. Safety of VBACs in birth centers: choices and risks. Birth 2005;32(3): 229–31.

58. Windrim R. Vaginal delivery in birth centre after previous caesarean section. Lancet 2005;365(9454):106–7.

59. Macdorman MF, Declercq E, Menacker F, et al. Neonatal mortality for low-risk women by method of delivery. Birth 2007;34(1):101–2.

60. Smith GC, Pell JP, Cameron AD, et al. Risk of perinatal death associated with labor after previous cesarean delivery in uncomplicated term pregnancies. JAMA 2002;287(20):2684–90.

61. Leung AS, Farmer RM, Leung EK, et al. Risk factors associated with uterine rupture during trial of labor after cesarean delivery: a case-control study. Am J Obstet Gynecol 1993;168(5):1358–63.

62. Avery MD, Carr CA, Burkhardt P. Vaginal birth after cesarean section: a pilot study of outcomes in women receiving midwifery care. J Midwifery Womens Health 2004;49(2):113–7.

63. Kobelin CG. Intrapartum management of vaginal birth after cesarean section. Clin Obstet Gynecol 2001;44(3):588–93.

64. Devoe LD, Croom CS, Youssef AA, et al. The prediction of "controlled" uterine rupture by the use of intrauterine pressure catheters. Obstet Gynecol 1992; 80(4):626–9.

65. Rodriguez MH, Masaki DI, Phelan JP, et al. Uterine rupture: are intrauterine pressure catheters useful in the diagnosis? Am J Obstet Gynecol 1989; 161(3):666–9.

66. Brown HC, Paranjothy S, Dowswell T, et al. Package of care for active management in labour for reducing caesarean section rates in low-risk women. Cochrane Database Syst Rev 2008;4:CD004907.

67. Berghella V, Baxter JK, Chauhan SP. Evidence-based labor and delivery management. Am J Obstet Gynecol 2008;199(5):445–54.

68. Albers LL. The evidence for physiologic management of the active phase of the first stage of labor. J Midwifery Womens Health 2007;52(3):207–15.

69. Simkin P, Bolding A. Update on nonpharmacologic approaches to relieve labor pain and prevent suffering. J Midwifery Womens Health 2004;49(6):489–504.

70. Simkin PP, O'hara M. Nonpharmacologic relief of pain during labor: systematic reviews of five methods. Am J Obstet Gynecol 2002;186(5 Suppl Nature): S131–59.

71. Smith CA, Collins CT, Cyna AM, et al. Complementary and alternative therapies for pain management in labour. Cochrane Database Syst Rev 2006;4:CD003521.

72. Alfirevic Z, Devane D, Gyte GM. Continuous cardiotocography (CTG) as a form of electronic fetal monitoring (EFM) for fetal assessment during labour. Cochrane Database Syst Rev 2006;3:CD006066.

73. Smyth RM, Alldred SK, Markham C. Amniotomy for shortening spontaneous labour. Cochrane Database Syst Rev 2007;4:CD006167.

74. McNiven PS, Williams JI, Hodnett E, et al. An early labor assessment program: a randomized, controlled trial. Birth 1998;25(1):5–10.

75. Sanchez-Ramos L, Bernstein S, Kaunitz AM. Expectant management versus labor induction for suspected fetal macrosomia: a systematic review. Obstet Gynecol 2002;100(5 Pt 1):997–1002.

76. Sakala C, Corry M. Evidence-based maternity care: what it is and what it can achieve. New York: Milbank Memorial Fund; 2008.
77. Brancato RM. A meta-analysis of passive descent versus immediate pushing in nulliparous women with epidural analgesia in the second stage of labor. J Obstet Gynecol Neonatal Nurs 2008;37(1):4–12.
78. Frigoletto FD Jr, Lieberman E, Lang JM, et al. A clinical trial of active management of labor. N Engl J Med 1995;333(12):745–50.
79. Selin L, Almstrom E, Wallin G, et al. Use and abuse of oxytocin for augmentation of labor. Acta Obstet Gynecol Scand 2009;88(12):1352–7.
80. Wei SQ, Luo ZC, Qi HP, et al. High-dose vs low-dose oxytocin for labor augmentation: a systematic review. Am J Obstet Gynecol 2010;203(4):296–304.
81. Jackson DJ, Lang JM, Ecker J, et al. Impact of collaborative management and early admission in labor on method of delivery. J Obstet Gynecol Neonatal Nurs 2003;32(2):147–57 [discussion: 158–60].
82. Chaillet N, Dumont A. Evidence-based strategies for reducing cesarean section rates: a meta-analysis. Birth 2007;34(1):53–64.
83. MacDorman MF, Singh GK. Midwifery care, social and medical risk factors, and birth outcomes in the USA. J Epidemiol Community Health 1998;52(5):310–7.
84. Cahill AG, Waterman BM, Stamilio DM, et al. Higher maximum doses of oxytocin are associated with an unacceptably high risk for uterine rupture in patients attempting vaginal birth after cesarean delivery. Am J Obstet Gynecol 2008; 199(1):32, e1–5.
85. Friedman EA. Classic pages in obstetrics and gynecology. The graphic analysis of labor. Emanuel A. Friedman. Am J Obstet Gynecol 1978;132(7):822–3.
86. Neal JL, Lowe NK, Patrick TE, et al. What is the slowest-yet-normal cervical dilation rate among nulliparous women with spontaneous labor onset? J Obstet Gynecol Neonatal Nurs 2010;39(4):361–9.
87. Khan KS, Rizvi A. The partograph in the management of labor following cesarean section. Int J Gynaecol Obstet 1995;50(2):151–7.
88. Lavender T, Alfirevic Z, Walkinshaw S. Effect of different partogram action lines on birth outcomes: a randomized controlled trial. Obstet Gynecol 2006;108(2): 295–302.
89. Rosenblatt RA, Dobie SA, Hart LG, et al. Interspecialty differences in the obstetric care of low-risk women. Am J Public Health 1997;87(3):344–51.
90. Jackson DJ, Lang JM, Swartz WH, et al. Outcomes, safety, and resource utilization in a collaborative care birth center program compared with traditional physician-based perinatal care. Am J Public Health 2003;93(6):999–1006.
91. Hatem M, Sandall J, Devane D, et al. Midwife led versus other models of care for childbearing women. Cochrane Database Syst Rev 2008;4:CD004667.
92. Harrington LC, Miller DA, McClain CJ, et al. Vaginal birth after cesarean in a hospital-based birth center staffed by certified nurse-midwives. J Nurse Midwifery 1997;42(4):304–7.
93. American College of Nurse-Midwives. Philosophy of the American College of Nurse-Midwives. Available at: http://www.midwife.org/philosophy.cfm. Accessed January 11, 2011.

The Influence of Intrapartum Factors on Risk of Uterine Rupture and Successful Vaginal Birth After Cesarean Delivery

Rosalie M. Grivell, BSc, BMBS*, Merlyn P. Barreto, MD,
Jodie M. Dodd, PhD, CMFM

KEYWORDS

* Cesarean delivery * VBAC * Uterine rupture * Vaginal birth

Cesarean delivery is one of the most common operative procedures performed worldwide, with the proportion of women giving birth by cesarean delivery increasing over the past several decades. The Australian data indicate an increase in cesarean delivery rates from 21.0% in 1998 to 30.9% in 2007.[1] Rates of cesarean birth have similarly increased in the United States, that is, from 20.7% of all births in 1996 to 31.1% in 2006.[2] The data from the United Kingdom indicate a similar trend, and although the overall rate of cesarean birth is lower at almost 25% of all births in 2007 to 2008, this rate has increased by almost 50% as per the data obtained in 1995 to 1996.[3] Reported cesarean delivery rates vary considerably across Europe, from 15% in Norway and the Netherlands to approximately 17% in Sweden and Finland, further increasing to 37.8% in Italy.[4] Cesarean birth rates approach 50% in many private hospitals in Chile, Argentina, Brazil, and Paraguay.[5]

There is considerable variability reported in the chance of a woman successfully achieving a vaginal birth after cesarean birth (VBAC), ranging between 56% and 80%, although there is far greater regional variation in the proportion of women who attempt VBAC.[6–10] For example, data from the United Kingdom indicate that among

The authors have nothing to disclose.
Discipline of Obstetrics and Gynaecology, The University of Adelaide, Women's and Children's Hospital, 72 King William Road, North Adelaide, South Australia 5006, Australia
* Corresponding author.
E-mail address: rosalie.grivell@adelaide.edu.au

Clin Perinatol 38 (2011) 265–275
doi:10.1016/j.clp.2011.03.006
0095-5108/11/$ – see front matter Crown Copyright © 2011 Published by Elsevier Inc. All rights reserved.

women who have had a previous cesarean delivery, the proportion of women being offered a trial of labor varied from 6% to 64% across institutions.[11] In contrast, data from sub-Saharan Africa indicate that the rates of planned VBAC are up to 97% (range 54%–97%), with 63% to 84% successful vaginal births.[12]

Although rates of cesarean birth have increased, there has been a concomitant reduction in the proportion of women who underwent a prior cesarean delivery and attempt a trial of labor in a subsequent pregnancy. The US data indicate that the rate of VBAC has declined from 28.3% in 1996 to 12.7% in 2002[13] and further to 8.3% in 2007.[14] Literature reports of seemingly increased maternal and infant health risks after VBAC, including uterine rupture[15–17] and perinatal death,[18] have not facilitated changes to clinical practice or public perception.

A prior cesarean birth is associated with a well-documented risk of uterine rupture after labor in a subsequent pregnancy.[19–22] Although the reported prevalence of uterine rupture among women who had a prior cesarean delivery is 1% worldwide, it is estimated that in developing countries, uterine rupture contributes up to 10% of maternal deaths.[23] The risks associated with attempted VBAC, particularly uterine scar rupture and perinatal death, are greater in cases in which the trial of labor is unsuccessful, and a cesarean delivery is required as an emergency procedure.[19–22] Consideration of factors during labor that may alter a woman's chances of successful VBAC is therefore of relevance, potentially allowing the identification of women for whom the chance of successful VBAC is low and therefore potentially associated with an increased risk of maternal and infant morbidity.

Although several tools have been described in the literature that identify clinical factors and scoring models to predict successful VBAC, the purpose of this review is to focus on the evidence relating to the effect of intrapartum factors on both the success of VBAC and the uterine rupture. These intrapartum factors include cervical factors (specifically cervical dilatation, effacement, Bishop score, and cervical position), the need for induction or augmentation of labor, the use of epidural analgesia, and fetal heart rate monitoring during labor. The current evidence for the influence of these factors on VBAC success and uterine rupture is considered, both individually and in the context of screening or prediction tools.

CERVICAL FACTORS AND THE CHANCE OF SUCCESSFUL VBAC

Cervical factors such as dilatation, effacement, and Bishop score are often used alone or in combination as an indicator of cervical favorability, all being associated with the likelihood of successful trial of labor. Each factor may be assessed in late pregnancy, at the time of the onset of spontaneous labor, or before commencing the process of induction of labor.

Cervical dilatation in late gestation has been consistently reported to be associated with the chance of successful VBAC, the presence of cervical dilatation increasing the chance of achieving vaginal birth.[24–28]

In a study of more than 5000 women undergoing trial of labor after a prior cesarean delivery, Flamm and Geiger[24] used logistic regression techniques to examine a variety of factors to evaluate their role in the prediction of successful VBAC. For women who were assessed after spontaneous onset of labor and found to have cervical dilatation larger than 4 cm, the chance of successful VBAC was 86%. In contrast, for women who at the time of admission had a cervical dilatation of less than 4 cm, the chance of successful VBAC decreased to 67% (adjusted relative risk [RR] was 2.16 for successful VBAC; 95% confidence interval [CI], 1.66–2.82).[24,29]

These findings have been subsequently confirmed by others.[25,26] Using data from the Maternal-Fetal Medicine Units Cesarean Registry, Landon and colleagues[26] examined factors influencing the success of a trial of labor, involving more than 14,000 women. Women who successfully achieved a VBAC were almost twice as likely to have evidence of cervical dilatation beyond 4 cm at the time of presentation of spontaneous labor or at the time of rupture of membranes when compared with women who did not achieve vaginal birth (48.1% vs 26.4%, $P<.001$).[26]

Similarly, Gonen and colleagues[25] report outcomes from a trial of labor involving 475 women who had a prior cesarean delivery. The presence of cervical dilatation at the time of presentation in labor significantly increased the likelihood of successfully achieving vaginal birth (odds ratio [OR], 2.5; 95% CI, 1.3–4.9).[25]

The presence of cervical effacement, whether measured at the time of admission in spontaneous labor[24] or at the time of commencing the process of induction of labor,[30] is associated with an increase in the chance of successful VBAC. In Flamm and Geiger's[24] prospective cohort, a cervical effacement of more than 25% was associated with an increased chance of a woman achieving vaginal birth when compared with a cervical effacement less than 25% (RR, 1.79; 95% CI, 1.31–2.44). The retrospective study by McNally and Turner[30] on birth outcomes in 103 women who had a previous cesarean delivery undergoing induction of labor indicated that a 100% cervical effacement at the time of commencing induction of labor was associated with a 5 times increased chance of successful VBAC (adjusted RR, 5.0; 95% CI, 1.28–19.2).

It is well recognized that the state of the cervix relates directly to the duration of pregnancy; this finding was first described by Bishop[31] in 1964, who published a quantitative pelvic scoring system based on 500 consecutive vaginal examinations performed on multiparous women who entered labor spontaneously after 36 weeks' gestation. The use of a modified Bishop score accounts for both cervical dilatation and effacement, as well as other features, including cervical position, consistency, and position of the fetal presenting part in relation to the maternal ischial spines.

In a retrospective cohort study, Bujold and colleagues[32] evaluated the outcomes in 685 women who had a previous cesarean delivery and required induction of labor. The chance of successful VBAC was significantly correlated with the modified Bishop score at time of commencing induction, with a score of more than 6 increasing the likelihood of vaginal birth (adjusted RR, 2.07; 95% CI, 1.28–3.35).[32] Similarly, other investigators have reported that a low Bishop score necessitating cervical ripening[33] or induction of labor in the presence of an unfavorable cervix[34] reduces the chance of vaginal birth while increasing the chance of cesarean birth.

CERVICAL FACTORS AND THE RISK OF UTERINE RUPTURE

Although there seems to be a relationship between cervical state and the chance of successful VBAC, any association between cervical favorability and the risk of uterine rupture remains less certain. In a small case-control study, a low Bishop score necessitating cervical ripening was reported to be a risk factor for uterine rupture.[35] However, in larger cohorts, uterine rupture does not seem to be associated with either Bishop score or other measures of an "unfavorable" cervix.[32–34] However, the available sample size of several of these studies[33,36] may well be underpowered to detect differences in an uncommon outcome. As discussed subsequently, it remains unclear if the observed increased risk of maternal morbidity and, in particular, uterine rupture in women with an unfavorable cervix reflects the need for induction of labor or whether it represents a specific effect modulated by changes in connective tissue structure after the use of prostaglandin preparations.

INDUCTION OF LABOR AND THE CHANCE OF SUCCESSFUL VBAC

Women who had a previous cesarean delivery and do not enter labor spontaneously may require cervical ripening and/or induction of labor depending on their cervical status. Although it may be ideal to avoid induction of labor in women who had a prior cesarean delivery, this either may become necessary, following the development of pregnancy complications, including postterm pregnancy,[30] or may be preferable to performing an elective repeat cesarean procedure.[37]

The reported chance of achieving a successful vaginal birth for women with a previous scar after induction of labor ranges from 51% to 80%.[30,33,38–40]

Landon and colleagues[26] reported the outcomes of more than 14,000 women who had a prior cesarean delivery who underwent a trial of labor in a subsequent pregnancy. In a secondary analysis of this data, induction of labor of any type was associated with a 50% reduction in the chance of a woman achieving a successful vaginal birth (OR for successful VBAC, 0.50; 95% CI, 0.45–0.55).[26] Among women who successfully achieved vaginal birth, 24.5% required induction of labor, compared with 34.2% of women who attempted vaginal birth but required cesarean birth.[26]

Similar findings were reported by Grobman and colleagues[39] in a prospective cohort study of 11,778 women who had a prior cesarean birth. Women who required induction of labor were less likely to achieve vaginal birth compared with women who entered labor spontaneously (51% vs 65%, $P<.001$).[39] Although women with a previous vaginal birth were more likely to achieve VBAC, the need for induction of labor remained associated with a statistically significant reduction in success compared with spontaneous onset of labor (83% vs 88%, $P<.001$).[39]

Rageth and colleagues[41] conducted a retrospective cohort study involving 29,000 women who had a prior cesarean birth. Again, women who required emergency cesarean birth were more likely to have required induction of labor when compared with women who successfully achieved VBAC (RR, 1.47; 95% CI, 1.37–1.59).[41]

INDUCTION OF LABOR AND THE RISK OF UTERINE RUPTURE

The risk of uterine rupture after induction of labor in women who had a prior cesarean delivery is well documented, with rates consistently reported to be greater (1.4%–2.3%) than those in women who enter labor spontaneously (0.45%–0.7%).[38,40,42,43]

In a population-based cohort study of 20,095 women with a first singleton birth by cesarean delivery, the trial of labor in a subsequent birth was associated with a significant increase in the risk of uterine rupture, which was 3-fold higher in women after spontaneous labor (RR, 3.3; 95% CI, 1.8–6.0), increasing further to between 5- and 15-fold after induction of labor, particularly with the administration of prostaglandin preparations.[16]

These findings are consistent with those reported by Landon and colleagues.[19] Although the overall risk of symptomatic uterine rupture among all women undergoing trial of labor was low at 0.7%, the risk was significantly increased among women who underwent induction of labor (48/4708 women; OR, 2.86; 95% CI, 1.75–4.67).[19] In a separate analysis, Grobman and colleagues[39] reported an increased risk of uterine rupture after induction of labor only among women who did not undergo a prior vaginal delivery (1.5% vs 0.8%, $P = .02$).

There is currently limited information available from randomized controlled trials evaluating specific methods of induction of labor for women who had a prior cesarean birth. The authors have identified 3 systematic reviews[44–46] that have included 4 randomized trials assessing different methods of induction of labor in this clinical setting. The combined sample size was 137 women, and because the methods of induction that were adopted in each individual trial varied considerably, it was not possible to incorporate the findings in a meta-analysis. Recommendations regarding the method of induction of labor in women who had a prior cesarean birth must therefore be based on available evidence of lower methodological quality.

Prostaglandin Induction of Labor

Prostaglandin E_2 and prostaglandin E_1 (including misoprostol) are commonly used for cervical ripening and induction of labor. Physiologically, prostaglandins act to increase the content of water, glycosaminoglycan levels, and hyaluronic acid levels in cervical tissue, with the resultant effect of an increasingly disorganized and pliable network of collagen fibers.[47,48] Although the local effect of prostaglandin preparations on cervical ripening is advantageous, systemic absorption also occurs, and a similar effect on connective tissue at other sites in the body, including uterine scar tissue, could potentially reduce strength and predispose to disruption or clinical rupture.

When compared with women with a uterine scar who enter labor spontaneously, prostaglandin induction of labor is associated with an increased risk of rupture.[16,19,49]

As indicated previously, the population-based study by Lydon-Rochelle and colleagues[16] identified a marked 4.7-fold increase in the risk of uterine rupture after prostaglandin administration for induction of labor. Similarly, Landon and colleagues[19] identified the use of prostaglandin preparations to be associated with an increased risk of uterine rupture (13/926 women; OR, 3.95; 95% CI, 2.01–7.79), when compared with women who entered labor spontaneously.

In contrast, Smith and colleagues[49] report Scottish data involving more than 36,000 women who had a prior cesarean birth, of whom 4600 underwent prostaglandin induction in a subsequent pregnancy. In this population-based study, the reported risk of uterine rupture and subsequent perinatal death after prostaglandin induction of labor was 11 per 10,000 labors compared with 4.5 per 10,000 labors in the absence of prostaglandin induction.[49] Induction of labor with prostaglandins was associated with almost a 50% increase in a woman's chance of emergency cesarean birth when compared with a woman whose labor was not induced (OR, 1.42; 95% CI, 1.26–1.60; $P<.001$).[49]

In all of the reported studies, although the RR of uterine rupture is increased after prostaglandin induction of labor, the absolute risk for any individual woman remains low.

Oxytocin

Zelop and colleagues[50] conducted a retrospective study involving 2775 women. After controlling for a variety of potential confounders, the risk for uterine rupture in women undergoing oxytocin labor induction was reported to be increased by 4.6-fold compared with the risk in women who entered labor spontaneously (rate of uterine rupture 2.0% vs 0.7%). Similarly, Landon and colleagues[19] reported a 3-fold increase in the risk of uterine rupture when labor was induced with oxytocin alone when compared with spontaneous onset of labor (OR, 3.01; 95% CI, 1.66–5.46; $P<.001$). In this study, the absolute risk of uterine rupture was 1.1%.

In contrast, Macones and colleagues[20] reported no increase in the risk of uterine rupture when oxytocin alone was used for induction of labor. However, although the use of prostaglandin preparations alone was not associated with an increased risk of uterine rupture, the sequential use of prostaglandins followed by oxytocin did seem to be associated with an increase in the risk of uterine rupture (adjusted OR, 3.07; 95% CI, 0.98–9.88).[20]

The effect of oxytocin dose, the regimen used, and the duration of administration during labor have all been implicated in the risk of uterine rupture. Although Goetzl and colleagues[51] failed to identify an association between oxytocin dosing regimen and total dose administered and the risk of uterine rupture, this has not been universally reported. In contrast, Cahill and colleagues[52] identified a relationship between oxytocin dose and risk of uterine rupture among women with a history of previous cesarean delivery. Within a nested case-control study of 804 women who had a prior cesarean delivery, 272 women were exposed to oxytocin. Of those women administered oxytocin, 62 were identified with a uterine rupture. In this study, maximum doses administered more than 20 mU/min increased the risk of uterine rupture by at least 4-fold (21–30 mU/min; hazard ratio, 3.92; 95% CI, 1.06–14.52).[52]

Mechanical Methods of Induction of Labor

There is a paucity of high-quality information describing mechanical methods of labor induction for women who had a previous cesarean delivery. Although the use of a transcervical Foley catheter (or other devices designed for this purpose) has been shown to be an effective cervical ripening agent, most studies included in the meta-analysis excluded women who had a prior cesarean delivery.[53]

Two retrospective studies have evaluated the use of mechanical methods of cervical ripening in women who had a prior cesarean birth. Bujold and colleagues' study of 2493 women who had a prior cesarean delivery reported a significant reduction in the VBAC success rate, which was 78% for women in spontaneous labor compared with 55.7% for women whose labor was induced by mechanical dilatation.[36] Ravasia and colleagues[43] examined rates of uterine rupture with different methods of induction of labor in 2119 women and reported only 1 case of uterine rupture in 149 women when an intracervical catheter was used for induction. Despite small numbers, this low rate of rupture was not significantly different when compared with uterine rupture rates after spontaneous labor.

Although both of these studies suggest that the use of mechanical cervical dilatation among women who had a prior cesarean birth is not associated with an increased risk of uterine rupture when compared with women who enter labor spontaneously,[36,43] this may be at the expense of a reduced chance of successful vaginal birth.

A small randomized controlled trial involving 213 women evaluated the role of serial membrane sweeping at term for women who were planning VBAC.[54] In this trial, membrane sweeping was not associated with an effect on the duration of pregnancy, the onset of labor, need for induction of labor, or risk of a repeat cesarean birth.[54] Although there were no adverse outcomes reported, the sample size is small and therefore is not powered to identify differences in rare clinical outcomes, including risk of uterine rupture.

AUGMENTATION OF LABOR

There is considerable controversy regarding the use of oxytocin, both to induce and augment labor in women with a scarred uterus. The use of oxytocin to augment labor has been repeatedly associated with a reduction in the chance of a woman achieving vaginal birth.[19,28,29,41,55] In their systematic review and meta-analysis, Eden and colleagues[29] report a reduction of 48% in the chance of successful VBAC after the use of oxytocin for augmentation of labor (OR, 0.52; 95%, CI 0.38–0.83).

As detailed previously, there is an increased risk of uterine rupture associated with the use of oxytocin for induction of labor, although it is less clear if this risk also extends to women undergoing augmentation of labor. Oxytocin augmentation is reported to increase the risk of uterine rupture by a factor of almost 2.5 times by some investigators,[19,29] increasing to 12.7-fold by others.[56] However, this finding is not uniform, with Rageth and colleagues[41] failing to identify an association between augmentation of labor and risk of uterine rupture.

EPIDURAL ANESTHESIA

There is no conclusive evidence of an effect of epidural analgesia on VBAC success rates in women who had a previous cesarean delivery. Two small retrospective studies (including <500 women) have reported a reduction in the chance of successful VBAC after the use of epidural analgesia.[25,30] In contrast, however, the larger National Institute of Child Health and Human Development cohort study by Landon and colleagues did not confirm this association,[26] and in fact, women who used epidural analgesia were more likely to successfully achieve vaginal birth (OR, 0.37; 95% CI, 0.33–0.41).[26]

Any association between the use of epidural analgesia and the risk of uterine rupture is uncertain. Although concern has been raised that the use of an epidural may mask a woman's experience of pain in the region of the uterine scar, which is considered to herald imminent uterine rupture, any causative effect remains tenuous. Rageth and colleagues[41] identified that among women who experienced uterine rupture, epidural analgesia was used 3 times more frequently than in women who did not have uterine rupture (RR, 2.88; 95% CI, 1.86–4.46). A more accurate indicator of impending uterine rupture may be an increasingly frequent need for analgesia or epidural "top-up," as indicated by Cahill and colleagues,[52] with a dose-response relationship evident between the number of epidural doses administered and risk of uterine rupture.

FETAL HEART RATE STATUS

Although the use of continuous electronic fetal heart rate monitoring in labor is often recommended for women attempting a VBAC,[11] its value in the management of labor in this setting is controversial.

Several studies have examined fetal heart rate patterns before uterine rupture.[41,57,58] Nonreassuring fetal heart rate tracing, particularly significant variable decelerations or fetal bradycardia, have been reported to be the most common finding accompanying uterine rupture.[16]

Results from the large cohort study by Rageth and colleagues[41] suggest that nonreassuring fetal heart rate status is associated with failed trial of labor; this outcome is noted twice as often in women with a failed trial of labor compared with those with successful VBAC (RR, 2.58; 95% CI, 2.35–2.83). In the same study, nonreassuring fetal heart rate status was also associated with uterine rupture (RR, 3.85, 95% CI, 2.67–5.55).[11]

A case-control study of 26 patients with uterine rupture found that both mild and severe variable fetal heart rate decelerations, especially in the presence of persistent abdominal pain, may predict uterine rupture in patients attempting VBAC. At less than 2 hours before delivery or acute uterine rupture, mild and severe variable decelerations, persistent abdominal pain, and uterine hyperstimulation were more common in these patients when compared with controls, and these patients had statistically significant positive likelihood ratios.[57] However, another case-control study with 36 cases of uterine rupture suggested that fetal bradycardia in the first and second stage is the only finding to differentiate uterine rupture from successful VBAC, with no significant differences identified in the occurrence of mild or severe variable decelerations, late decelerations, prolonged decelerations, fetal tachycardia, or loss of uterine tone.[58]

A systematic review by Guise and colleagues[59] on the incidence and consequences of uterine rupture in women who had a previous cesarean delivery reported that despite the presence of adequate personnel to proceed with emergency cesarean delivery, prompt intervention does not always prevent fetal neurologic injury.

PREDICTIVE TOOLS

As indicated earlier, a range of intrapartum factors may influence a woman's chance of successful vaginal birth and risk of uterine rupture in the setting of a prior cesarean birth. In particular, the spontaneous onset of labor and more advanced cervical dilatation at the time of admission to hospital in labor or at the time of rupture of membranes are both significantly associated with successful VBAC and a decreased risk of uterine rupture, in contrast to the effects of requiring either induction or augmentation of labor.

In an attempt to identify women with a higher chance of successful VBAC and an acceptably low risk of uterine rupture, many investigators have developed screening tools to predict success and risk of complications. Those tools which use intrapartum factors, either alone or in combination with antepartum factors, are likely to be of the greatest value in a clinical setting; this type of combined screening tool allows a woman and her primary carer to assess the chance of successful VBAC early in pregnancy using identifiable factors and to then reassess these risks subsequently should induction or augmentation of labor be required. The description and evaluation of these predictive tools are beyond the scope of this article.

The recently published evidence report by Guise and colleagues[8] outlines a detailed description and evaluation of screening tools and other predictors of VBAC and uterine rupture for women undergoing VBAC. This comprehensive review highlights the screening tools by Flamm and Geiger,[24] Smith and colleagues,[49] and Grobman and colleagues[34] to be amongst the strongest tools available because the tools have been either externally validated or cross-validated by others. These investigators conclude that the models to predict VBAC that include intrapartum factors provide reasonable ability to identify women who have a reasonable chance of a successful VBAC, but none have discriminating ability to consistently identify women who are at risk for cesarean birth.[8]

SUMMARY

To date there is limited high-quality information to guide clinical decision making for women and their clinicians in the setting of a prior cesarean birth. Although the literature reports a woman's chance of successful VBAC to be relatively constant at 74%,[8] there is considerable variation in the proportion of women who attempt a trial of labor after cesarean delivery. The most consistently identified intrapartum factors associated with successful vaginal birth and lower risk of uterine rupture are the spontaneous onset of labor and advanced cervical dilatation, whether measured in late pregnancy, at the time of hospital admission in labor or membrane rupture, or before commencing induction of labor. In contrast, need for induction and augmentation of labor are both factors associated with an increased likelihood of failed trial of labor and risk of uterine rupture.

REFERENCES

1. Laws P, Sullivan EA. Australia's mothers and babies 2007. Perinatal statistics series No. 23 Cat. No. PER 48. Sydney (Australia): Australian National Perinatal STatistics Unit; 2009.

2. Martin JA, Hamilton BE, Sutton PD, et al. Births: final data for 2006, vol. 57. 7th edition. Hyattsville (MD): U.S. Department of Health and Human Services, National Center for Health Statistics, National Vital Statistics System; 2009.
3. HES Online. Hospital episode statistics. Method of delivery, 1980 to 2007–8. (UK): National Health Services; 2009.
4. Zeitlin J, Mohangoo A. European perinatal health report. Paris (France): EURO-Peristat Project; 2004.
5. Belizan JM, Althabe F, Barros FC, et al. Rates and implications of caesarean sections in Latin America: ecological study. BMJ 1999;319(7222):1397–400.
6. Appleton B, Targett C, Rasmussen M, et al. Vaginal birth after Caesarean section: an Australian multicentre study. VBAC Study Group. Aust N Z J Obstet Gynaecol 2000;40(1):87–91.
7. Flamm BL. Once a cesarean, always a controversy. Obstet Gynecol 1997;90(2): 312–5.
8. Guise JM, Eden K, Emeis C, et al. Vaginal birth after cesarean: new insights. Evid Rep Technol Assess (Full Rep) 2010;191(191):1–397.
9. McMahon MJ. Vaginal birth after cesarean. Clin Obstet Gynecol 1998;41(2): 369–81.
10. Stone C, Halliday J, Lumley J, et al. Vaginal births after Caesarean (VBAC): a population study. Paediatr Perinat Epidemiol 2000;14(4):340–8.
11. Thomas J, Paranjothy S. Royal College of Obstetricians and Gynaecologists Clinical Effectiveness Support Unit. The National Sentinel Caesarean Section Audit Report. London: RCOG Press; 2001.
12. Boulvain M, Fraser WD, Brisson-Carroll G, et al. Trial of labour after caesarean section in sub-Saharan Africa: a meta-analysis. Br J Obstet Gynaecol 1997; 104(12):1385–90.
13. Menacker F, Hamilton BE. Recent trends in cesarean delivery in the United States. NCHS Data Brief 2010;35(35):1–8.
14. Martin JA, Hamilton BE, Ventura SJ. Births: final data for 2007. Natl Vital Stat Rep 2010;57(12):1–23.
15. Hibbard JU, Ismail MA, Wang Y, et al. Failed vaginal birth after a cesarean section: how risky is it? I. Maternal morbidity. Am J Obstet Gynecol 2001; 184(7):1365–71 [discussion: 1371–3].
16. Lydon-Rochelle M, Holt VL, Easterling TR, et al. Risk of uterine rupture during labor among women with a prior cesarean delivery. N Engl J Med 2001;345(1):3–8.
17. Sachs BP, Kobelin C, Castro MA, et al. The risks of lowering the cesarean-delivery rate. N Engl J Med 1999;340(1):54–7.
18. Smith GC, Pell JP, Cameron AD, et al. Risk of perinatal death associated with labor after previous cesarean delivery in uncomplicated term pregnancies. JAMA 2002;287(20):2684–90.
19. Landon MB, Hauth JC, Leveno KJ, et al. Maternal and perinatal outcomes associated with a trial of labor after prior cesarean delivery. N Engl J Med 2004; 351(25):2581–9.
20. Macones GA, Peipert J, Nelson DB, et al. Maternal complications with vaginal birth after cesarean delivery: a multicenter study. Am J Obstet Gynecol 2005; 193(5):1656–62.
21. McMahon MJ, Luther ER, Bowes WA Jr, et al. Comparison of a trial of labor with an elective second cesarean section. N Engl J Med 1996;335(10):689–95.
22. Rossi AC, D'Addario V. Maternal morbidity following a trial of labor after cesarean section vs elective repeat cesarean delivery: a systematic review with metaanalysis. Am J Obstet Gynecol 2008;199(3):224–31.

23. Hofmeyr GJ, Say L, Gulmezoglu AM. WHO systematic review of maternal mortality and morbidity: the prevalence of uterine rupture. BJOG 2005;112(9): 1221–8.
24. Flamm BL, Geiger AM. Vaginal birth after cesarean delivery: an admission scoring system. Obstet Gynecol 1997;90(6):907–10.
25. Gonen R, Tamir A, Degani S, et al. Variables associated with successful vaginal birth after one cesarean section: a proposed vaginal birth after cesarean section score. Am J Perinatol 2004;21(8):447–53.
26. Landon MB, Leindecker S, Spong CY, et al. The MFMU Cesarean Registry: factors affecting the success of trial of labor after previous cesarean delivery. Am J Obstet Gynecol 2005;193(3 Pt 2):1016–23.
27. Learman LA, Evertson LR, Shiboski S. Predictors of repeat cesarean delivery after trial of labor: do any exist? J Am Coll Surg 1996;182(3):257–62.
28. Macones GA, Hausman N, Edelstein R, et al. Predicting outcomes of trials of labor in women attempting vaginal birth after cesarean delivery: a comparison of multivariate methods with neural networks. Am J Obstet Gynecol 2001; 184(3):409–13.
29. Eden KB, McDonagh M, Denman MA, et al. New insights on vaginal birth after cesarean: can it be predicted? Obstet Gynecol 2010;116(4):967–81.
30. McNally OM, Turner MJ. Induction of labour after 1 previous Caesarean section. Aust N Z J Obstet Gynaecol 1999;39(4):425–9.
31. Bishop EH. Pelvic scoring for elective induction. Obstet Gynecol 1964;24:266–8.
32. Bujold E, Blackwell SC, Hendler I, et al. Modified Bishop's score and induction of labor in patients with a previous cesarean delivery. Am J Obstet Gynecol 2004; 191(5):1644–8.
33. Grinstead J, Grobman WA. Induction of labor after one prior cesarean: predictors of vaginal delivery. Obstet Gynecol 2004;103(3):534–8.
34. Grobman WA, Lai Y, Landon MB, et al. Development of a nomogram for prediction of vaginal birth after cesarean delivery. Obstet Gynecol 2007;109(4):806–12.
35. Weimar CH, Lim AC, Bots ML, et al. Risk factors for uterine rupture during a vaginal birth after one previous caesarean section: a case-control study. Eur J Obstet Gynecol Reprod Biol 2010;151(1):41–5.
36. Bujold E, Blackwell SC, Gauthier RJ. Cervical ripening with transcervical Foley catheter and the risk of uterine rupture. Obstet Gynecol 2004;103(1):18–23.
37. Dodd J, Crowther CA. Vaginal birth after Caesarean section: a survey of practice in Australia and New Zealand. Aust N Z J Obstet Gynaecol 2003;43(3):226–31.
38. Delaney T, Young DC. Spontaneous versus induced labor after a previous cesarean delivery. Obstet Gynecol 2003;102(1):39–44.
39. Grobman WA, Gilbert S, Landon MB, et al. Outcomes of induction of labor after one prior cesarean. Obstet Gynecol 2007;109(2 Pt 1):262–9.
40. Zelop CM, Shipp TD, Cohen A, et al. Trial of labor after 40 weeks' gestation in women with prior cesarean. Obstet Gynecol 2001;97(3):391–3.
41. Rageth JC, Juzi C, Grossenbacher H. Delivery after previous cesarean: a risk evaluation. Swiss Working Group of Obstetric and Gynecologic Institutions. Obstet Gynecol 1999;93(3):332–7.
42. Chilaka VN, Cole MY, Habayeb OM, et al. Risk of uterine rupture following induction of labour in women with a previous caesarean section in a large UK teaching hospital. J Obstet Gynaecol 2004;24(3):264–5.
43. Ravasia DJ, Wood SL, Pollard JK. Uterine rupture during induced trial of labor among women with previous cesarean delivery. Am J Obstet Gynecol 2000; 183(5):1176–9.

44. Dodd JM, Crowther CA. Vaginal birth after caesarean versus elective repeat caesarean for women with a single prior caesarean birth: a systematic review of the literature. Aust N Z J Obstet Gynaecol 2004;44(5):387–91.
45. National Collaborating Centre for Women's and Children's Health. Induction of labour—clinical guideline. London (UK): RCOG Press; 2008.
46. McDonagh MS, Osterweil P, Guise JM. The benefits and risks of inducing labour in patients with prior caesarean delivery: a systematic review. BJOG 2005;112(8): 1007–15.
47. Danforth DN, Veis A, Breen M, et al. The effect of pregnancy and labor on the human cervix: changes in collagen, glycoproteins, and glycosaminoglycans. Am J Obstet Gynecol 1974;120(5):641–51.
48. Uldbjerg N, Ekman G, Malmstrom A, et al. Ripening of the human uterine cervix related to changes in collagen, glycosaminoglycans, and collagenolytic activity. Am J Obstet Gynecol 1983;147(6):662–6.
49. Smith GC, White IR, Pell JP, et al. Predicting cesarean section and uterine rupture among women attempting vaginal birth after prior cesarean section. PLoS Med 2005;2(9):e252.
50. Zelop CM, Shipp TD, Repke JT, et al. Outcomes of trial of labor following previous cesarean delivery among women with fetuses weighing >4000 g. Am J Obstet Gynecol 2001;185(4):903–5.
51. Goetzl L, Shipp TD, Cohen A, et al. Oxytocin dose and the risk of uterine rupture in trial of labor after cesarean. Obstet Gynecol 2001;97(3):381–4.
52. Cahill AG, Waterman BM, Stamilio DM, et al. Higher maximum doses of oxytocin are associated with an unacceptably high risk for uterine rupture in patients attempting vaginal birth after cesarean delivery. Am J Obstet Gynecol 2008; 199(1):32. e31–5.
53. Boulvain M, Kelly A, Lohse C, et al. Mechanical methods for induction of labour. Cochrane Database Syst Rev 2001;4:CD001233.
54. Hamdan M, Sidhu K, Sabir N, et al. Serial membrane sweeping at term in planned vaginal birth after cesarean: a randomized controlled trial. Obstet Gynecol 2009; 114(4):745–51.
55. Spaans WA, Sluijs MB, van Roosmalen J, et al. Risk factors at caesarean section and failure of subsequent trial of labour. Eur J Obstet Gynecol Reprod Biol 2002; 100(2):163–6.
56. Dekker GA, Chan A, Luke CG, et al. Risk of uterine rupture in Australian women attempting vaginal birth after one prior caesarean section: a retrospective population-based cohort study. BJOG 2010;117(11):1358–65.
57. Craver Pryor E, Mertz HL, Reaver BW, et al. Intrapartum predictors of uterine rupture. Am J Perinatol 2007;24(5):317–21.
58. Ridgeway JJ, Weyrich DL, Benedetti TJ. Fetal heart rate changes associated with uterine rupture. Obstet Gynecol 2004;103(3):506–12.
59. Guise JM, McDonagh MS, Osterweil P, et al. Systematic review of the incidence and consequences of uterine rupture in women with previous caesarean section. BMJ 2004;329(7456):19–25.

Uterine Rupture During a Trial of Labor After Previous Cesarean Delivery

Carolyn M. Zelop, MD*

KEYWORDS

- Uterine rupture • Trial of labor after previous cesarean
- Risk factors • Protective factors

Controversy surrounding a trial of labor (TOL) in women with a history of prior cesarean delivery has been dominated by the fear of uterine rupture. Although the overall risk of uterine rupture is less than 1%,[1] the potential for maternal and neonatal morbidity and even mortality remain paramount concerns for both patients and health care providers. In a study encompassing 142,075 women undergoing a TOL after previous cesarean birth, the uterine rupture–related complication rate per 1000 TOL's was 1.8 for maternal transfusion, 1.5 for fetal acidosis less than 7.0, 0.8 for genitourinary injury, 0.4 for perinatal death, and 0.02 for maternal death.[2] Before embarking on a discussion of prevalence rates of uterine rupture and variables that may modify these risks, it is important to establish a working definition. The recent National Institutes of Health (NIH) Consensus Development Conference entitled "Vaginal Birth after Cesarean: New Insights" defined uterine rupture as the complete anatomic separation of the uterine wall regardless of the presence or absence of symptoms with or without extrusion of the fetal-placental unit.[3] Although uterine dehiscence, which implies an incomplete disruption of the uterine wall with intact serosa, may be clinically relevant as a near-miss uterine rupture, the rates of the 2 entities will not be used interchangeably. However, some studies choose to report these together as disruptions of normal uterine anatomy.

Although the rates differ among various cohorts, the literature consistently reports an increased risk of uterine rupture in women undergoing a TOL compared with elective repeat cesarean delivery (ERCD). According to the NIH Consensus Statement,[3] the risk of uterine rupture for women of all gestational ages undergoing a TOL is 0.33%

The author has nothing to disclose.
Beth Israel Deaconess Medical Center, Division of Maternal Fetal Medicine, Harvard University School of Medicine, Boston, MA 02215, USA
* Beth Israel Deaconess Medical Center, 330 Brookline, KS 338, Boston, MA 02215.
E-mail address: cmzelop@comcast.net

Clin Perinatol 38 (2011) 277–284
doi:10.1016/j.clp.2011.03.009
0095-5108/11/$ – see front matter © 2011 Elsevier Inc. All rights reserved.

compared with 0.03% for women undergoing ERCD. At term, the risk of uterine rupture is 0.78% in women undergoing TOL compared with 0.02% in those undergoing ERCD. Perhaps the most clinically relevant analyses are based on intention to deliver.[4] Spong and colleagues[5] stratified the analysis of uterine rupture among 39,117 women at term with a history of cesarean delivery by 5 subgroups that might be encountered by the clinician including (1) TOL (n = 15,323), (2) ERCD with labor (n = 2721), (3) ERCD without labor (n = 14,993), (4) indicated repeat cesarean delivery with labor (n = 1078), and (5) indicated repeat cesarean delivery without labor (n = 5002). In this study, the rate of uterine rupture in women who underwent TOL was 0.74% in contrast to those who underwent ERCD with or without labor, who sustained a rate of 0.15% and 0%, respectively. The group with indicated repeat cesarean delivery with or without labor experienced slightly higher rates of uterine rupture compared with the group with ERCD (0.28% and 0.08%, respectively).

FACTORS AFFECTING THE INTEGRITY OF THE HYSTEROTOMY SCAR

There is a paucity of data regarding wound healing of the hysterotomy scar. Various modalities including radiological and pathologic studies as well as an animal model have been used to gain insight, yet information remains sparse.[6–8] Wound healing is characterized as an initial inflammatory process with recruitment of fibroblasts and synthesis of collagen to create a scar matrix. Theoretically, remodeling of the initial uterine hysterotomy scar under the influence of growth factors, such as insulinlike growth factor 1, might favor the eventual regeneration of the myometrium.[6] Using ultrasonography to evaluate the appearance of both single- and double-layer closure of the hysterotomy, Hamar and colleagues[8] demonstrated an initial increase in the thickness of the postpartum uterus that was 5- to 6-fold at 48 hours after delivery. Although there was a gradual decrease in the uterine thickness over the 6-week course, the uterine scar thickness remained increased compared with the predelivery baseline irrespective of the mode of hysterotomy closure technique suggesting ongoing scar remodeling after the traditional postpartum period. The small sample size may have precluded the detection of an observed difference in the thickness between the closure techniques. However, magnetic resonance imaging has suggested that remodeling and restoration of the uterine zonal anatomy in a lower transverse hysterotomy lasts at least 6 months.[7]

Factors affecting the integrity of the hysterotomy scar may modify the risk of uterine rupture during a TOL after previous cesarean birth. Shipp and colleagues[9] demonstrated that postpartum fever, which could impede the healing process of the hysterotomy scar complicating the index cesarean birth, is associated with an increased risk of uterine rupture during a subsequent TOL. A short interdelivery interval that does not allow enough time for complete hysterotomy healing may be associated with an increased risk of uterine rupture during a TOL after previous cesarean.[10,11] An interdelivery interval of less than or equal to 18 months is associated with a 3-fold increased risk of uterine rupture during a subsequent TOL after previous cesarean birth.[10] The technique of prior uterine closure (single- vs double-layer suturing of the hysterotomy) has also been studied as a possible risk factor for uterine rupture. Although results have been inconsistent in the literature, the largest study to date by Bujold and colleagues[12] demonstrated an almost 3-fold increased risk of uterine rupture during TOL after previous cesarean birth when single-layer closure of the hysterotomy was used in the index pregnancy. Further analysis in this study revealed no association between uterine rupture and suture material used for hysterotomy closure. Other factors not well studied because of sample size include other aspects of surgical technique, such as interlocking suture placement. Complicating the concept of tensile strength of the repaired hysterotomy governing the chance of uterine rupture during TOL after previous cesarean is the documentation of uterine rupture remote from the lower uterine segment.[13]

CLINICAL FACTORS THAT MODIFY THE RISK OF UTERINE RUPTURE DURING TOL

Clinical research initiated in the late 1990s, which continued into the new millennium, identified factors that increase or decrease the risk of uterine rupture during a TOL after previous cesarean. Identifying women with the least risk of uterine rupture should potentially optimize the safety of vaginal birth after cesarean (VBAC). Both antepartum and intrapartum factors should be considered.

UTERINE SCAR TYPE AND NUMBER OF PRIOR CESAREAN DELIVERIES

Most of the literature examining outcomes of TOL has focused on women with prior low transverse hysterotomy, and indeed, this cohort has become the referent group in other comparative studies.[4] In the largest study examining women with prior low vertical hysterotomy undergoing TOL after previous cesarean birth, Shipp and colleagues[14] demonstrated a 0.8% risk of symptomatic uterine rupture, which was not increased when compared with those with a prior low transverse uterine incision. This study had a power of 80% to detect an increase from 1% (as noted for low transverse incisions) to 3% risk of symptomatic uterine rupture, which has been observed in women undergoing a TOL after multiple previous cesarean births.

Recent studies have reported a range of risk of uterine rupture from 0.9% to 3.7% during a TOL after 2 prior cesareans compared with a TOL after single prior cesarean birth,[15–17] leading to some inconsistencies in the interpretation of the data. Although there is an increased risk of major maternal morbidity associated with TOL after more than 1 prior cesarean delivery, the absolute risk remains small. All 3 studies suggested a protective effect of prior vaginal delivery when undergoing a TOL after more than 1 prior cesarean birth.

DEMOGRAPHIC CHARACTERISTICS, PRIOR OBSTETRIC HISTORY, AND THE RISK OF UTERINE RUPTURE

More recently, demographic factors have been demonstrated to influence the risk of uterine rupture, and because these factors can be identified in the antepartum period, they can be used for counseling women. In a retrospective cohort study, Shipp and colleagues[18] demonstrated that increasing maternal age was associated with a greater chance of uterine rupture. In this study, women younger than 30 years undergoing a TOL after previous cesarean delivery had a 0.5% risk of uterine rupture compared with a risk of 1.4% in those aged 30 years or older. Age, in general, seems to hinder abdominal wound healing, and it also seems to affect uterine hysterotomy healing in a model controlling for other risk factors that modify the risk of uterine rupture. Any previous vaginal delivery is associated with a decreased risk of uterine rupture during a TOL after previous cesarean birth. Using a logistic regression model controlling for possible confounders such as epidural analgesia, year of birth, maternal age, birthweight, duration of labor, and use of oxytocin for augmentation or induction, Zelop and colleagues[19] demonstrated that women with a previous vaginal delivery experienced one-fifth the risk (0.2% vs 1.1%) of uterine rupture during a TOL after previous cesarean when compared with women without prior vaginal delivery.

Fetal size and maternal body mass index (BMI), defined as the weight in kilograms divided by the height in meters squared, seem to have some influence on the risk of uterine rupture during a TOL after previous cesarean birth. Birthweight is used as a proxy for estimated fetal weight in the literature when examining the risk of uterine rupture. Zelop and colleagues[20] reported no statistically increased risk of uterine rupture among women with fetuses weighing more than 4000 g compared with those weighing 4000 g or less during a TOL after previous cesarean. Caution was recommended for fetuses with birthweights less than 4250 g because the rate of rupture was 2.4% in this group of women undergoing a TOL after previous cesarean. Elkousy and colleagues[21] concluded in their analysis that women with no prior vaginal deliveries and neonatal birthweight greater than or equal to 4000 g were at an increased risk of uterine rupture with a rate of 3.6%. Increasing BMI also seems to increase the risk of uterine rupture and dehiscence. The combined risk increased from 0.9% to 2.1% when comparing women with a normal BMI undergoing a TOL after previous cesarean with morbidly obese women defined as those with a BMI greater than 40.[22]

Gestational age of the current pregnancy may influence the risk of uterine rupture. Compared with women with term pregnancies undergoing a TOL after previous cesarean birth, those laboring preterm seem to have lower rates of uterine rupture (0.34% vs 0.74%).[23] For spontaneous labor, uterine rupture during a TOL after the estimated day of delivery (EDD) seems to be similar to the risk before EDD as reported in 2 cohort studies.[24,25] If the previous cesarean delivery was preterm, the risk for uterine rupture in the subsequent TOL is minimally increased when compared with the risk in women who had previous term cesarean deliveries. In a multivariable analysis controlling for confounders, patients with a previous preterm cesarean delivery remained at an increased risk of subsequent uterine rupture during a TOL when compared with women with previous term cesarean delivery with an odds ratio of 1.6 corresponding to an absolute increased risk from 0.68% to 1.0%.[26]

LABOR MANAGEMENT AND THE RISK OF UTERINE RUPTURE

Discussion of induction and augmentation of labor after previous cesarean birth is a broad topic that is covered in depth in an article by Grivell and colleagues elsewhere in this issue. Therefore, the discussion in this article revolves around the effect of induction and augmentation on the risk of uterine rupture during a TOL after previous cesarean birth. Induction of labor with oxytocin is associated with an increased risk of uterine rupture. Zelop and colleagues[27] demonstrated an overall rate of uterine rupture of 2.3% among patients with induction of labor compared with 0.7% among women with spontaneous labor. In a logistic regression model controlling for possible confounders, induction of labor in women with prior cesarean and no other deliveries was associated with a 4.6-fold increased risk of uterine rupture. In this same model, there was a trend toward increased risk of uterine rupture associated with use of prostaglandin E_2 gel, although this difference was not statistically different. In a subsequent study to further clarify the effect of prostaglandin use, Lydon-Rochelle and colleagues[28] confirmed the increased risk of induction compared with repeated cesarean delivery and demonstrated the highest risk associated with use of prostaglandins particularly misoprostol. Landon and colleagues[29] reported a statistically significant increased risk of uterine rupture associated with induction of labor after previous cesarean delivery regardless of the method used compared with spontaneous labor after previous cesarean birth.

Variable results have been reported regarding the association of augmentation of labor and the risk of uterine rupture during a TOL after previous cesarean birth. Goetzl and colleagues[30] demonstrated no differences in exposure to oxytocin between cases defined as women with uterine rupture who received oxytocin and controls defined as women who received oxytocin and sustained no uterine rupture. In contrast, Landon and colleagues[29] reported a 0.9% risk of uterine rupture in women receiving oxytocin for augmentation of labor compared with 0.4% in women with spontaneous labor after previous cesarean delivery. In addition, Cahill and colleagues[31] demonstrated a statistically significant 4-fold or greater increased risk of uterine rupture when maximum dosages greater than 20 mU/min of oxytocin were used for augmentation of labor during a TOL after previous cesarean birth.

PREDICTION OF UTERINE RUPTURE

Can uterine rupture be predicted in women attempting a TOL after previous cesarean birth? Ideally, the most suitable candidates for a TOL after previous cesarean have the lowest risk of uterine rupture and the highest chance of a successful vaginal delivery. Two approaches have been explored in the literature for the prediction of uterine rupture: assessment of the lower uterine segment (LUS) and prediction nomograms or multivariable models.

Rozenberg and colleagues[32] evaluated a transabdominal ultrasonographic approach to assess the thickness of the LUS in patients with a history of prior cesarean at 36to 38 weeks as a screening tool to predict the risk of intrapartum uterine rupture. Their technique performed with a full bladder seemed to measure the thinnest portion of the myometrium in the LUS. Analysis of their data demonstrated that the risk of a defective scar was related to thinning of the LUS as measured by ultrasonography. Using a cutoff of 3.5 mm, the sensitivity of the ultrasonographic measurement was 88%, with a positive predictive value of 11.8% but a negative predictive value of 99.3%. Using these data, women with an LUS greater than or equal to 3.5 mm may be considered for a TOL after previous cesarean birth. Subsequently, Bujold and colleagues[33] demonstrated that a full LUS thickness of less than 2.3 mm is associated with a higher risk of complete uterine rupture. A recent systematic review of the use of sonographic LUS thickness in predicting uterine scar defect demonstrated that although LUS thickness is a strong predictor for uterine scar disruption, no ideal cutoff has been identified.[34] More studies are required before this tool is ready for widespread clinical use because the technical aspects of its reproducibility have yet to be validated and would require large-scale monitoring similar to nuchal translucency measurement in practice.

Several multivariable models have been proposed in the literature as well. Macones and colleagues[35] investigated the use of both antepartum and early labor factors to develop a model predictive of uterine rupture. Their study using receiver operating characteristic curves, which examined such factors including prior vaginal delivery, ethnicity, maternal age, gestational age, induction of labor, and cervical dilation greater than 3 cm, failed to achieve sensitivity and specificity that are clinically useful. Grobman and colleagues[36] sought to develop a model that predicted individual specific risk for uterine rupture. They divided their data into a training set and a testing set. The logistic regression model that yielded the optimal final prediction tool failed to achieve discriminating ability necessary to predict uterine rupture that was clinically useful. Lastly, Shipp and colleagues[37] proposed an assessment tool for prediction of intrapartum uterine rupture based on factors available early in the antepartum period. Using their scoring system based on 40 symptomatic uterine ruptures and 4384 TOL's, 60% of uterine ruptures would be prevented while allowing 81% of patients a TOL. About 36 elective repeat cesarean deliveries would be performed to prevent 1 symptomatic uterine rupture. Although this model seemed to perform well and the sample size was robust, it was not large enough to enable a validation phase to be performed. Thus, in summary, although several reasonable models have been designed to predict uterine rupture, prospective studies are required to continue to optimize their clinical utility for the satisfactory prediction of uterine rupture during a TOL after previous cesarean birth.

SUMMARY

Uterine rupture, which involves complete separation of the uterine wall, occurs in about 1% of those attempting VBAC. Because uterine rupture is one of the most significant complications of a TOL after previous cesarean, identifying those at increased risk of uterine rupture is paramount to the safety of a TOL after previous cesarean birth. It seems that both antepartum demographic characteristics and intrapartum factors modify the risk of uterine rupture. The ability to reliably predict an individual's a priori risk for intrapartum uterine rupture remains a major area of investigation.

REFERENCES

1. Fang YM, Zelop CM. Vaginal birth after cesarean: assessing maternal and perinatal risks-contemporary management. Clin Obstet Gynecol 2006;49:147–53.
2. Chauhan SP, Martin JN, Henrichs CE, et al. Maternal and perinatal complications with uterine rupture in 142,075 patients who attempted vaginal birth after cesarean delivery: a review of the literature. Am J Obstet Gynecol 2003;189: 408–17.
3. NIH Consensus Development Conference on Vaginal Birth After Cesarean: New Insights. March 8–10, 2010. Available at: http://concensus.nih.gov/2010/images/vbac/vbac_statement.pdf. Accessed August 23, 2010.
4. American College of Obstetricians and Gynecologists. Vaginal birth after previous cesarean delivery. Practice bulletin No. 115. Obstet Gynecol 2010; 116:450–63.
5. Spong CY, Landon MB, Gilbert S, et al. Risk of uterine rupture and adverse perinatal outcome at term after cesarean delivery. Obstet Gynecol 2007;110:801–7.
6. Bowers D, McKenzie D, Dutta D, et al. Growth hormone treatment after cesarean delivery in rats increases the strength of the uterine scar. Am J Obstet Gynecol 2001;185:614–7.
7. Dicle O, Kucukler C, Pinar T, et al. Magnetic resonance imaging evaluation of incision healing after cesarean sections. Eur Radiol 1997;7(1):31–4.
8. Hamar B, Saber S, Cackovic, et al. Ultrasound evaluation of the uterine scar after cesarean delivery: a randomized controlled trial of one and two layer closure. Obstet Gynecol 2007;110:808–13.
9. Shipp TD, Zelop CM, Cohen A, et al. Post-cesarean delivery fever and uterine rupture in a subsequent trial of labor. Obstet Gynecol 2003;101:136–9.
10. Shipp TD, Zelop CM, Repke JT, et al. Interdelivery interval and risk of symptomatic uterine rupture. Obstet Gynecol 2001;97:175–7.
11. Bujold E, Gauthier RJ. Risk of uterine rupture associated with an interdelivery interval between 18-24 weeks. Obstet Gynecol 2010;115(5):1003–6.
12. Bujold E, Goyet M, Marcoux S, et al. The role of uterine closure in the risk of uterine rupture. Obstet Gynecol 2010;116:43–50.
13. Buhimschi CS, Buhimschi SP, Malinow A, et al. Rupture of the uterine scar during term labour: contractility or biochemistry? BJOG 2005;112(1):38–42.

14. Shipp TD, Zelop CM, Repke JT, et al. Intrapartum uterine rupture and dehiscence in patients with prior lower uterine segment vertical and transverse incisions. Obstet Gynecol 1999;94:735–40.
15. Landon MB, Spong CY, Thom E, et al. Risk of uterine rupture with a trial of labor in women with multiple and single prior cesarean delivery. Obstet Gynec 2006; 108(1):12–20.
16. Macones GA, Cahill A, Pare E, et al. Obstetric outcomes in women with two prior cesarean deliveries: is vaginal birth after cesarean delivery a viable option? Am J Obstet Gynecol 2005;192:1223–9.
17. Caughey AB, Shipp TD, Repke JT, et al. Rate of uterine rupture during a trial of labor in women with one or two prior cesarean deliveries. Am J Obstet Gynecol 1999;181:872–6.
18. Shipp TD, Zelop CM, Repke JT, et al. The association of maternal age and symptomatic uterine rupture during a trial of labor after prior cesarean delivery. Obstet Gynecol 2002;99:585–8.
19. Zelop CM, Shipp TD, Repke JT, et al. Effect of previous vaginal delivery on the risk of uterine rupture during a subsequent trial of labor. Am J Obstet Gynecol 2000;183:1184–6.
20. Zelop CM, Shipp TD, Repke JT, et al. Outcomes of trial of labor following previous cesarean delivery among women with fetuses weighing >4000g. Am J Obstet Gynecol 2001;185(4):903–5.
21. Elkousy MA, Sammel M, Stevens E, et al. The effect of birth weight on vaginal birth after cesarean delivery success rates. Am J Obstet Gynecol 2003;188: 824–30.
22. Hibbard JU, Gilbert S, Landon MB, et al. Trial of labor or repeat cesarean delivery in women with morbid obesity and previous cesarean delivery. Obstet Gynecol 2006;108:125–33.
23. Durnwald CP, Rouse DJ, Leveno KL, et al. The maternal-fetal medicine units cesarean registry: safety and efficacy of a trial of labor in preterm pregnancy after a prior cesarean delivery. Am J Obstet Gynecol 2006;195(4):1119–26.
24. Zelop CM, Shipp TD, Cohen A, et al. Trial of labor after 40 weeks' gestation in women with prior cesarean. Obstet Gynecol 2001;97(3):391–3.
25. Coassolo KM, Stamilio DM, Pare E, et al. Safety and efficacy of vaginal birth after cesarean attempts at or beyond 40 weeks' of gestation. Obstet Gynecol 2005; 106(4):700–6.
26. Sciscione AC, Landon MB, Leveno KJ, et al. Previous preterm cesarean delivery and risk of subsequent uterine rupture. Obstet Gynecol 2008;111(3):648–53.
27. Zelop CM, Shipp TD, Repke JT, et al. Uterine rupture during induced or augmented labor in gravid women with one prior cesarean delivery. Am J Obstet Gynecol 1999;181:882–6.
28. Lydon-Rochelle M, Holt VL, Easterling TR, et al. Risk of uterine rupture during labor among women with a prior cesarean delivery. N Engl J Med 2001; 345(1):3–8.
29. Landon MB, Hauth JC, Leveno KJ, et al. Maternal and perinatal outcomes associated with a trial of labor after prior cesarean delivery. N Engl J Med 2004;351: 2581–9.
30. Goetzl L, Shipp TD, Cohen A, et al. Oxytocin dose and the risk of uterine rupture in trial of labor after cesarean. Obstet Gynecol 2001;97:381–4.
31. Cahill AG, Waterman BM, Stamilio DM, et al. Higher maximum doses oxytocin are associated with unacceptably high risk for uterine rupture in patients attempting vaginal birth after cesarean delivery. Am J Obstet Gynecol 2008;199:32.e1–5.

32. Rozenberg P, Goffinet F, Philippe HJ, et al. Ultrasonographic measurement of lower uterine segment to assess risk of defects of scarred uterus. Lancet 1996; 347:281–4.
33. Bujold E, Jastrow N, Simoneau J, et al. Prediction of complete uterine rupture by sonographic evaluation of the lower uterine segment. Am J Obstet Gynecol 2009; 201(3):320.e1–6.
34. Jastrow N, Chaillet N, Roberge S, et al. Sonographic lower uterine segment thickness and the risk of uterine scar defect: a systematic review. J Obstet Gynaecol Can 2010;32(4):321–7.
35. Macones G, Cahill AG, Stamilio AM, et al. Can uterine rupture in patients attempting vaginal birth after cesarean delivery be predicted? Am J Obstet Gynecol 2006;195:1148–52.
36. Grobman WA, Lei Y, Landon MB, et al. Prediction of uterine rupture associated with attempted vaginal birth after cesarean delivery. Am J Obstet Gynecol 2008;199:30.e1–5.
37. Shipp TD, Zelop CM, Lieberman E. Assessment of the rate of uterine rupture at the first prenatal visit: a preliminary evaluation. J Maternal Fetal Neonatal Med 2008;21(2):129–33.

Multiple Repeat Cesareans and the Threat of Placenta Accreta: Incidence, Diagnosis, Management

Andrew D. Hull, MD[a], Thomas R. Moore, MD[b],*

KEYWORDS

• Placenta accreta • Cesarean section • Incidence
• Management

At the time of writing, a third of women delivering in the United States of America do so by cesarean section.[1] The rates of both primary and repeat cesarean section have risen steadily in the last few decades and show no sign of flattening off. The increase in primary cesarean rate reflects increased rates of maternal obesity, increased numbers of multiple gestations secondary to assisted reproductive technology, physician concern about litigation for adverse obstetric outcome,[1] and a decline in the use of operative vaginal delivery for both cephalic and breech presentations.[2] The increase in repeat cesarean section rate reflects a move away from the use of trial of labor after cesarean section (TOLAC) and a consequent decrease in the rate of vaginal birth after cesarean section (VBAC). The decline in VBAC numbers has attracted much recent attention and is the focus of an ongoing process to remedy the situation.[3,4] Nonetheless, it is likely that, despite these efforts, there will continue to be further increases in the overall cesarean section rate in the future.

With the background of increasing numbers of cesarean delivery, women are also undergoing repetitive cesarean sections. Such multiple surgical procedures are becoming increasingly common and have consequences for both short-term care and long-term complications.[5,6] Perhaps the most pressing complication associated

The authors have nothing to disclose.
a Division of Perinatal Medicine, Department of Reproductive Medicine, University of California San Diego, 200 West Arbor Drive #8433, La Jolla, San Diego, CA 92103-8433, USA
b Department of Reproductive Medicine, University of California San Diego, 200 West Arbor Drive #8433, La Jolla, San Diego, CA 92103-8433, USA
* Corresponding author.
E-mail address: trmoore@ucsd.edu

Clin Perinatol 38 (2011) 285–296
doi:10.1016/j.clp.2011.03.010
0095-5108/11/$ – see front matter © 2011 Elsevier Inc. All rights reserved.

with prior cesarean delivery is the occurrence of placenta accreta.[7] Placenta accreta is defined as an abnormal adherence of the placenta to the uterine wall. It has traditionally been classified as placenta accreta, placenta increta, and placenta percreta based on how deeply the placenta is attached to the myometrium: superficial, deep, and through to serosa and adjacent structures, respectively. Because management is similar for all grades of abnormal attachment, the term placenta accreta is used here to cover all these possibilities. In cases of placenta accreta, the placenta fails to separate normally after delivery of the infant and results in primary postpartum hemorrhage that is often worsened by attempts to remove the placenta, producing a horrifying spiral of hemorrhage, coagulopathy, and shock.

INCIDENCE

Placenta accreta complicates about 3 per 1000 deliveries in the United States.[7] This represents a substantial increase in incidence compared with the rates of around 1 per 10,000 seen in the 1960s,[8] and reflects a tripling of incidence since the 1980s. The most important factor in this increase is the increase in incidence of cesarean section. Placenta accreta remains a rare occurrence in the unscarred uterus.[5] Although cases have been reported following prior myomectomy, curettage, or treatment of Asherman syndrome, the prevailing risk factor for accreta is the presence of a uterine scar from prior cesarean section.

In women undergoing primary cesarean section for indications other than placenta previa, the incidence of placenta accreta is around 0.03%. A second or subsequent cesarean section without placenta previa is associated with an increase in the risk of accreta that rises with each subsequent cesarean section. For a second to a fifth cesarean section, the incidence remains less than 1%, although an increase to 4.7% is observed at the sixth and subsequent procedures (**Fig. 1**).[5]

A further risk factor for placenta accreta is placenta previa. Placenta previa affects about 0.5% of all pregnancies at term.[9] This number rises to as high as 5% in pregnancies in which a prior cesarean section was performed.[10,11] Again, with increasing number of prior cesarean sections, the risk of placenta previa proportionally increases.[12] In women undergoing primary cesarean section for placenta previa,

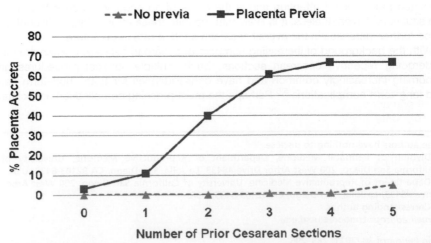

Fig. 1. Incidence of placenta accreta in women with prior cesarean section with and without coexisting placenta previa.

the incidence of placenta accreta is about 3.3%. The presence of a uterine scar significantly increases this risk; 1 prior cesarean section plus placenta previa is associated with a risk of placenta accreta of 11%, 2 prior cesarean sections a risk of 40%, 3 prior cesarean sections 61%, and 4 or more prior cesarean sections 67% (see **Fig. 1**).[5]

Because prior cesarean section is independently associated with an increased risk for placenta previa and placenta previa, the presence of a prior uterine scar is the most important factor in the observed dramatically increased incidence of placenta accreta.[13] It follows that any increase in repeat cesarean section rate and number of cesarean sections performed will increase the number of cases of placenta accreta that occur.

Other factors associated with an independent increase in the risk of placenta previa are increased maternal age (>35 years, ×5 increase in risk,[14] >40 years, ×90 increase in risk[10]). Such factors become additive as older women undergo more cesarean sections.

It is not known why a prior cesarean section increases the likelihood of placenta previa and why placenta accreta is so prevalent in cases of placenta previa with multiple prior cesarean sections. The uterus heals by secondary intention and it has been suggested that the scarred area fails to decidualize normally, leading to abnormal placentation and loss of the normal cleavage plane above the decidua basalis. Primary defects in trophoblast function with abnormal tissue invasion have also been suggested to play a role. The area of uterine scarring may be hypoxic, which may in turn be causative of both abnormal decidualization and trophoblast behavior.

It has been suggested that the widespread practice of single-layer uterine closure after cesarean section may lead to inadequate uterine healing and has contributed to the increase in the number of cases of placenta accreta. Choice of suture material may also play a part, with traditional chromic catgut producing suboptimal healing compared with synthetic suture material. There are no randomized studies addressing this issue, nor are animal studies available to support this contention; it remains an area in need of exploration.

DIAGNOSIS

The gold standard for diagnosis of placenta accreta is pathologic examination of the uterus and attached placenta. When multiple tissue sections are evaluated in cases undergoing hysterectomy, areas showing the full range of depth of invasion from accreta to increta, and sometimes percreta, often coexist. This finding supports a uniform approach to management of all cases regardless of apparent depth of invasion as assessed by antepartum imaging.

The primary screening tool for placenta accreta is ultrasound imaging. All women with placenta previa should be evaluated for abnormal placentation. Those with a history of prior cesarean section or other uterine scarring should be carefully evaluated for features suggesting placenta accreta.[7]

Localization of the placenta should be included in the anatomy scan between 18 and 20 weeks. Initial imaging should be transabdominal and those with an apparently low-lying placenta should be evaluated with transvaginal ultrasound. If a complete or partial placenta previa is identified, subsequent imaging is recommended at 28 to 32 weeks to evaluate the placental position and need for cesarean delivery.[7] The likelihood of persistence of placenta previa into the third trimester is increased by the degree of overlap of the cervix by the placenta[15–17] and the thickness of the placental edge.[18] All women who present with bleeding after 20 weeks' gestation should be evaluated for placenta previa; subsequent imaging and mode of delivery may be dictated by clinical presentation in such cases rather than absolute measurements of placental position. Typically, if the placenta is 2 to 2.5 cm from the internal os at 28 to 32 weeks, vaginal delivery should be possible without undue risk of bleeding.[19] If the placenta is less than 2 cm from the cervix at 28 to 32 weeks, further imaging at 34 weeks may identify cases with greater distance and thus permit vaginal delivery.

All cases of placenta previa should be regarded as being at risk for placenta accreta and the ultrasound features suggesting abnormal placentation looked for carefully. The mainstay of diagnosis is grayscale ultrasound, although color[20,21] and power Doppler and three-dimensional (3D) reconstruction[22] have been reported to be helpful in clarifying difficult cases. The ultrasound features suggesting placenta accreta are[23,24]:

1. Loss of echolucent area between the placenta and uterus
2. Multiple placental lacunae (Swiss-cheese appearance)
3. Loss of echolucent line between the placenta and bladder
4. Focal exophytic masses extending into the bladder
5. Color Doppler findings may include:
   - Vascular lakes with turbulent flow
   - Hypervascularity of serosa-bladder interface
   - Abnormal nonanatomic vessels bridging placental thickness
   - Diffuse or focal lacunar flow.
6. Power Doppler with 3D may show hypervascularity, abnormal coherent vessels in the serosa-bladder interface, and abnormal cotyledonal and intervillous circulations with chaotic branching and aberrant vessels.

Fig. 2 shows a recent case with features suggestive of placenta accreta. This woman had a complete placenta previa and history of 3 prior cesarean sections. Placenta percreta was confirmed at delivery.

A recent review[25] examined the performance of the different ultrasound modalities in diagnosing placenta accreta. Grayscale ultrasound had a sensitivity of 95% and a specificity of 76% for the diagnosis of accreta. Color Doppler gave values of 92% and 68% and 3D power Doppler 100% and 85%, respectively. The positive predictive

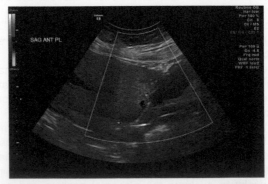

Fig. 2. Transabdominal ultrasound scan at 19 weeks showing complete placenta previa with loss of echolucent area between placenta and uterus anteriorly, loss of echolucent plane between bladder and placenta, and a bulge of placenta into bladder, all suggesting placenta accreta and possible percreta.

values were 82%, 76%, and 88% for each modality. In general, the more abnormal features that are seen, the greater the diagnostic accuracy.

Several investigators have evaluated the use of magnetic resonance imaging (MRI) in the diagnosis of placenta accreta.[26,27] To date, there are no generally agreed standards for MRI evaluation of suspected placenta accreta. Some authorities favor the use of gadolinium, whereas others do not routinely use contrast. The common MRI features suggesting placenta accreta are:

1. Uterine bulging, especially into the region of the scar or bladder
2. Heterogeneous signal intensity within the placenta
3. Dark intraplacental bands on T2-weighted imaging.

A typical MRI scan is shown in **Fig. 3** (the same case as seen in **Fig. 2**); the findings suggest placenta percreta with bladder involvement.

Most diagnostic paradigms rely on ultrasound for screening and initial evaluation of suspected cases of accreta, reserving MRI for cases in which ultrasound is inconclusive or placenta percreta is suspected to aid in surgical planning.[24,26] MRI may be more helpful in cases of posterior placenta previa because of the potential difficulty evaluating the posterior placenta with ultrasound late in gestation.

Additional clues to the presence of placenta accreta may be obtained from abnormalities in serum testing used for aneuploidy screening. Increased maternal serum α-fetoprotein[13,28] and human chorionic gonadotropin (hCG)[13] (values more than 2.5 multiples of the median) have each been found to be correlated with placental

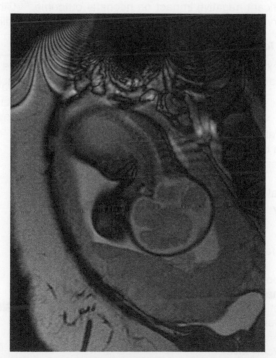

Fig. 3. MRI with gadolinium contrast at 30 weeks' gestational age for the same case as **Fig. 2.** Complete placenta previa with placenta percreta with possible blabber involvement; note bulging lower segment in region of bladder.

invasion, (odds ratio 8.3 and 3.9 respectively). These analyses have not been prospectively evaluated for predictive value or diagnostic thresholds set.

MANAGEMENT

Once the diagnosis of placenta accreta is established, a comprehensive written management plan needs to be accomplished. The key issues to be included are location and timing of delivery, multidisciplinary team care, the chosen surgical approach (hysterectomy or conservative management), and use of adjunctive treatments and techniques. A scheduled delivery is the goal because it is associated with the best outcome,[29,30] but a plan for intervention should the patient require earlier delivery for bleeding is also advised.[8]

Location and Timing of Delivery

Women should be scheduled for delivery at an appropriately equipped institution with adequate surgical resources and ready access to a blood bank that can supply the large amounts of blood products that may be needed. Typically, this is best accomplished in the setting of a tertiary center. The timing of elective delivery is important: too early and there is an undue risk of morbidity caused by prematurity, and too late increases the risk of hemorrhage and emergent delivery with consequent increases in mortality and morbidity. There are no prospective data to guide timing of delivery; however, a recent decision tree analysis favored delivery at 34 weeks' gestation after administration of antepartum steroids to improve fetal lung maturity.[31] It has been our practice to deliver patients at this gestational age after steroids for more than a decade without any significant negative impact on neonatal outcome.[30] Others have advocated later delivery at 36 weeks in women without a history of bleeding.[7]

Multidisciplinary Team Approach

Given the complexity and potential for disastrous outcome in these cases, we have recommended that care is provided by a multidisciplinary approach to include the following:

1. Team
   - Maternal-fetal medicine/obstetrics
   - Gynecologic oncology
   - Urology/other surgery
   - Anesthesia
   - Interventional radiology
   - Neonatology
   - Nursing
   - Social work
   - Patient and family.
2. Resources
   - Operating room
   - Inpatient rehabilitation suite
   - Postanesthetic care unit (PACU)/surgical intensive care unit (SICU)
   - Labor and delivery
   - Blood bank
   - Perfusionist/cell saver.

Others have also taken this approach with similar lists.[7,32,33] Eller and colleagues[32] compared the multidisciplinary approach with standard obstetric care in women with placenta accreta and found lower rates of early reoperation, transfusion volume, and overall morbidity in the multidisciplinary group.

Counseling and Coordination of Care

Following a confirmed diagnosis of placenta accreta, we recommend transfer of care to a tertiary care team. A critical part of that transfer of care is the establishment of a point person or individuals who will coordinate care and lead the formation and inter-action of the multidisciplinary team; in our institution this responsibility is assumed by a maternal-fetal medicine specialist.

Patient counseling is a critical part of the care process. Patients need to be given all relevant information early in the planning process and be aided in making informed decisions regarding their care. We favor elective cesarean hysterectomy as the safest approach to these patients, a view endorsed by others.[7,33] We do not offer conserva-tive or uterine preserving management in our center for patients with placenta previa accreta, and patients who desire such an approach receive appropriate counseling and referral to a center that chooses to provide such care as early in the management process as possible.

Timeline for Elective Delivery

Approximately 1 to 4 weeks before planned delivery by cesarean hysterectomy, we assemble the multidisciplinary team and lay out a discrete timeline for the individual patient's care. Patients visit the neonatal intensive care unit and labor and delivery unit 1 to 2 weeks before delivery and receive neonatology and anesthesiology consults. Two doses of betamethasone (12 mg intramuscularly 24 hours apart) are administered a week before delivery to help with fetal lung maturation. Patients are admitted the day before delivery and have laboratory work including crossmatching of blood products.

On the morning of delivery, an epidural may be placed to aid in the placement of internal iliac balloon catheters if required. Following this, the patient is transferred to the main operating room for placement of central venous access and arterial lines. Delivery may take place under epidural anesthesia or general anesthesia. Following delivery of the infant, all hysterectomies are performed under general anesthesia. Patients are recovered to PACU and typically spend 24 hours in SICU before transfer to labor and delivery.

Anesthetic Considerations

The choice of anesthetic technique should be made by the anesthesiologist respon-sible for the procedure. In the past, regional anesthesia has been favored for patients with placenta previa based on 2 small trials[34,35] in which blood loss and complications were more common in those receiving general anesthesia. Most hysterectomies for placenta accreta are performed under general anesthesia, and a case could easily be made for conducting both the delivery and the hysterectomy under the same anes-thetic. In the absence of evidence, either technique is acceptable. In either case, the most experienced anesthetist available should participate in these procedures.[33]

Surgical Approach

Patients may be positioned frog-legged to aid in visualization of intraoperative vaginal bleeding,[7] although this is not our routine practice. The surgical team should comprise the most able and experienced surgeons available. We believe that the combination of maternal-fetal medicine specialists and a gynecologic oncologist is optimal. Complex cases may require input from urologists and vascular and general surgery. The abdomen is usually opened through a vertical midline incision that can easily be extended to facilitate exposure. The uterus should be opened in the manner of a classic cesarean section, staying away from the placental implantation site; this may result in a transfundal incision. The baby is delivered and handed to the pediatric staff. No attempt is made to remove the placenta and uterotonics are not typically given because of the risk of partial placental separation and increased hemorrhage.[8,29] The uterus is whip stitched and the hysterectomy begun. We typically perform a posterior approach and a type II hysterectomy in which the ureters are carefully identified and preserved. The bladder flap is left until last in cases of anterior accreta; stringent efforts are made to avoid direct handling or dissection at the area of accreta. In many instances, a subtotal hysterectomy suffices.

Blood products

We recommend that women are crossmatched for 6 to 10 units of packed red blood cells and that 4 units of thawed fresh frozen plasma (FFP) are available together with a 10 pack of platelets. A massive transfusion protocol should be in place so that further blood products can be made available without delay in case of catastrophic hemorrhage. An excellent, comprehensive set of best practices for obstetric hemorrhage, including the components of an obstetric massive transfusion protocol, are freely available at the California Maternal Quality Care Collaborative Web site (www.cmqcc.org).

It is imperative that blood loss is actively managed and that early replacement takes place before coagulopathy develops in the setting of massive hemorrhage. Typically, platelets and FFP are given once a predefined amount (4–6 units) of packed red cells has been administered. Recent battlefield experience suggests that packed red blood cells and FFP should be given in a 1:1 ratio if large blood losses are encountered. This treatment results in reduced risk of coagulopathy, decreased need for postoperative transfusion, and decreased mortality.[36–38]

Recombinant factor VII has been used to treat massive bleeding from placenta accreta. Dosing ranges from 30 to 90 μg/kg and may be repeated in 2 to 3 hours. In extreme cases, it may be life saving,[39] although there seems to be a significant risk of thrombotic complications when it is used in the obstetric setting.[40,41]

The use of cell-saver autotransfusion seems to be safe in obstetric practice and free of the risk of amniotic fluid embolism.[42] However, it has not been widely adopted. There are no prospective studies of its use; in our own practice, we usually set up the device, although we have used it only rarely.

Adjunctive Aids to Surgery

Ureteric stents have been advocated as a useful aid to avoiding ureteric injury in these complex cases; there is only 1 retrospective study to date[29] and the data are inconclusive. However, it is difficult to imagine that their use would be harmful. Pelvic artery occlusion using balloon catheters has been advocated by several investigators, including ourselves.[8,30,43,44] Others have suggested that there is little overall effect on blood loss and that complications of catheter placement, including infection, thrombosis, and tissue necrosis, are unacceptable risks,[29,45,46] whereas others have reported mixed results.[47] We continue to place catheters before surgery in many cases, although we inflate the balloons during surgery in less than 20% of cases in response to severe hemorrhage. In this circumstance, we believe that the occlusive catheters are useful, although it is difficult to prove this. Both catheters and 1 sheath are removed after surgery in an attempt to reduce thrombotic complications. One sheath is left in place overnight to facilitate targeted embolization should secondary hemorrhage occur.

Prophylactic pelvic artery ligation has been suggested to be useful in this setting,[48] although Eller and colleagues[29] found it unhelpful in their series.

Postoperative Care/Complications

The most common complication encountered is postoperative bleeding. Patients should thus be monitored after surgery in an intensive care setting for the first postoperative day. Transfer to a step-down facility or labor and delivery unit is recommended for stable patients thereafter.

Emergent Cases

As previously stated, the outcomes for emergently managed cases are usually worse than those managed electively. A care plan with a protocol for emergent care should be part of all identified antenatal accreta cases. Much of the elective protocol can be applied to good effect.

Conservative Management

We believe that cesarean hysterectomy is the optimum management for all cases of placenta accreta, although we acknowledge that conservative management is an option favored by some. The principal reason for pursuing conservative treatment is the preservation of fertility; a less common indication would be placenta percreta not immediately amenable to definitive surgery because of operative difficulties or lack of resources. Conservative treatment includes stepwise uterine devascularization, intraoperative and postoperative embolization of pelvic vessels, methotrexate therapy, placental bed suturing, and intrauterine balloon occlusion. The latter 2 are unlikely to be successful except in cases of focal accreta, and may worsen outcome by delaying definitive surgery.

One recent review of 60 cases[49] managed conservatively had 26 cases in which the placenta was partially removed, 22 cases in which the placenta was left in situ and methotrexate given, and 12 cases in which the placenta was undisturbed and arterial embolization performed. Failure of treatment occurred in all 3 groups, with a secondary hysterectomy rate of 20%. Eleven women had serious infectious complications, 21 had significant vaginal bleeding, and 4 developed disseminated intravascular coagulation. Pregnancies occurred subsequently in 8 women. Another recent series[50] reported on 167 women with placenta accreta managed conservatively. Treatment was successful in 131/167 cases. Eighteen hysterectomies were performed for primary postpartum hemorrhage and 18 were done as delayed procedures for persistent hemorrhage, sepsis, and other morbidities. The investigators concluded that most patients with placenta accreta should be offered primary definitive surgery.

SUMMARY

Placenta accreta is a significant source of obstetric morbidity and mortality. Its incidence is increasing as a direct consequence of the increasing cesarean section rate. Optimum management for most cases requires elective cesarean hysterectomy, ideally performed at about 34 weeks' gestation. A multidisciplinary approach produces the best outcomes.

REFERENCES

1. Zhang J, Troendle J, Reddy UM, et al. Contemporary cesarean delivery practice in the United States. Am J Obstet Gynecol 2010;203(4):326, e1–326, e10.

2. Goetzinger KR, Macones GA. Operative vaginal delivery: current trends in obstetrics. Womens Health (Lond Engl) 2008;4(3):281–90.
3. ACOG Practice bulletin no. 115: vaginal birth after previous cesarean delivery. Obstet Gynecol 2010;116(2 Pt 1):450–63.
4. National Institutes of Health Consensus Development conference statement: vaginal birth after cesarean: new insights March 8–10, 2010. Obstet Gynecol 2010;115(6):1279–95.
5. Silver RM, Landon MB, Rouse DJ, et al. Maternal morbidity associated with multiple repeat cesarean deliveries. Obstet Gynecol 2006;107(6):1226–32.
6. Silver RM. Delivery after previous cesarean: long-term maternal outcomes. Semin Perinatol 2010;34(4):258–66.
7. Belfort MA. Placenta accreta. Am J Obstet Gynecol 2010;203(5):430–9.
8. Hull AD, Resnik R. Placenta accreta and postpartum hemorrhage. Clin Obstet Gynecol 2010;53(1):228–36.
9. Frederiksen MC, Glassenberg R, Stika CS. Placenta previa: a 22-year analysis. Am J Obstet Gynecol 1999;180(6 Pt 1):1432–7.
10. Ananth CV, Wilcox AJ, Savitz DA, et al. Effect of maternal age and parity on the risk of uteroplacental bleeding disorders in pregnancy. Obstet Gynecol 1996; 88(4 Pt 1):511–6.
11. Sheiner E, Shoham-Vardi I, Hallak M, et al. Placenta previa: obstetric risk factors and pregnancy outcome. J Matern Fetal Med 2001;10(6):414–9.
12. Grobman WA, Gersnoviez R, Landon MB, et al. Pregnancy outcomes for women with placenta previa in relation to the number of prior cesarean deliveries. Obstet Gynecol 2007;110(6):1249–55.
13. Hung TH, Shau WY, Hsieh CC, et al. Risk factors for placenta accreta. Obstet Gynecol 1999;93(4):545–50.
14. Iyasu S, Saftlas AK, Rowley DL, et al. The epidemiology of placenta previa in the United States, 1979 through 1987. Am J Obstet Gynecol 1993;168(5):1424–9.
15. Becker RH, Vonk R, Mende BC, et al. The relevance of placental location at 20-23 gestational weeks for prediction of placenta previa at delivery: evaluation of 8650 cases. Ultrasound Obstet Gynecol 2001;17(6):496–501.
16. Taipale P, Hiilesmaa V, Ylostalo P. Transvaginal ultrasonography at 18-23 weeks in predicting placenta previa at delivery. Ultrasound Obstet Gynecol 1998;12(6): 422–5.
17. Mustafa SA, Brizot ML, Carvalho MH, et al. Transvaginal ultrasonography in predicting placenta previa at delivery: a longitudinal study. Ultrasound Obstet Gynecol 2002;20(4):356–9.
18. Ghourab S. Third-trimester transvaginal ultrasonography in placenta previa: does the shape of the lower placental edge predict clinical outcome? Ultrasound Obstet Gynecol 2001;18(2):103–8.
19. Oyelese Y, Smulian JC. Placenta previa, placenta accreta, and vasa previa. Obstetrics and gynecology 2006;107(4):927–41.
20. Lerner JP, Deane S, Timor-Tritsch IE. Characterization of placenta accreta using transvaginal sonography and color Doppler imaging. Ultrasound Obstet Gynecol 1995;5(3):198–201.
21. Twickler DM, Lucas MJ, Balis AB, et al. Color flow mapping for myometrial invasion in women with a prior cesarean delivery. J Matern Fetal Med 2000;9(6): 330–5.
22. Chou MM, Tseng JJ, Ho ES, et al. Three-dimensional color power Doppler imaging in the assessment of uteroplacental neovascularization in placenta previa increta/percreta. Am J Obstet Gynecol 2001;185(5):1257–60.

23. Comstock CH. Antenatal diagnosis of placenta accreta: a review. Ultrasound Obstet Gynecol 2005;26(1):89–96.
24. Warshak CR, Eskander R, Hull AD, et al. Accuracy of ultrasonography and magnetic resonance imaging in the diagnosis of placenta accreta. Obstet Gynecol 2006;108(3 Pt 1):573–81.
25. Shih JC, Palacios Jaraquemada JM, Su YN, et al. Role of three-dimensional power Doppler in the antenatal diagnosis of placenta accreta: comparison with gray-scale and color Doppler techniques. Ultrasound Obstet Gynecol 2009; 33(2):193–203.
26. Levine D, Hulka CA, Ludmir J, et al. Placenta accreta: evaluation with color Doppler US, power Doppler US, and MR imaging. Radiology 1997;205(3):773–6.
27. Lam G, Kuller J, McMahon M. Use of magnetic resonance imaging and ultrasound in the antenatal diagnosis of placenta accreta. J Soc Gynecol Investig 2002;9(1):37–40.
28. Zelop C, Nadel A, Frigoletto FD Jr, et al. Placenta accreta/percreta/increta: a cause of elevated maternal serum alpha-fetoprotein. Obstet Gynecol 1992; 80(4):693–4.
29. Eller AG, Porter TF, Soisson P, et al. Optimal management strategies for placenta accreta. BJOG 2009;116(5):648–54.
30. Warshak CR, Ramos GA, Eskander R, et al. Effect of predelivery diagnosis in 99 consecutive cases of placenta accreta. Obstet Gynecol 2010;115(1):65–9.
31. Robinson BK, Grobman WA. Effectiveness of timing strategies for delivery of individuals with placenta previa and accreta. Obstet Gynecol 2010;116(4): 835–42.
32. Eller AG, Bennett MA, Sharshiner M, et al. Maternal morbidity in cases of placenta accreta managed by a multidisciplinary care team compared with standard obstetric care. Obstet Gynecol 2011;117(2 Pt 1):331–7.
33. Green-top Guideline No. 27 Placenta praevia, placenta praevia accreta and vasa praevia: diagnosis and management. London: RCOG; 2011. p.1–26.
34. Parekh N, Husaini SW, Russell IF. Caesarean section for placenta praevia: a retrospective study of anaesthetic management. Br J Anaesth 2000;84(6):725–30.
35. Hong JY, Jee YS, Yoon HJ, et al. Comparison of general and epidural anesthesia in elective cesarean section for placenta previa totalis: maternal hemodynamics, blood loss and neonatal outcome. Int J Obstet Anesth 2003;12(1):12–6.
36. Gonzalez EA, Moore FA, Holcomb JB, et al. Fresh frozen plasma should be given earlier to patients requiring massive transfusion. J Trauma 2007;62(1):112–9.
37. Holcomb JB, Wade CE, Michalek JE, et al. Increased plasma and platelet to red blood cell ratios improves outcome in 466 massively transfused civilian trauma patients. Ann Surg 2008;248(3):447–58.
38. Gunter OL Jr, Au BK, Isbell JM, et al. Optimizing outcomes in damage control resuscitation: identifying blood product ratios associated with improved survival. J Trauma 2008;65(3):527–34.
39. Pepas LP, Arif-Adib M, Kadir RA. Factor VIIa in puerperal hemorrhage with disseminated intravascular coagulation. Obstet Gynecol 2006;108(3 Pt 2): 757–61.
40. Alfirevic Z, Elbourne D, Pavord S, et al. Use of recombinant activated factor VII in primary postpartum hemorrhage: the Northern European registry 2000–2004. Obstet Gynecol 2007;110(6):1270–8.
41. Franchini M, Franchi M, Bergamini V, et al. A critical review on the use of recombinant factor VIIa in life-threatening obstetric postpartum hemorrhage. Semin Thromb Hemost 2008;34(1):104–12.

42. Catling SJ, Williams S, Fielding AM. Cell salvage in obstetrics: an evaluation of the ability of cell salvage combined with leucocyte depletion filtration to remove amniotic fluid from operative blood loss at caesarean section. Int J Obstet Anesth 1999;8(2):79–84.

43. Bodner LJ, Nosher JL, Gribbin C, et al. Balloon-assisted occlusion of the internal iliac arteries in patients with placenta accreta/percreta. Cardiovasc Intervent Radiol 2006;29(3):354–61.

44. Shih JC, Liu KL, Shyu MK. Temporary balloon occlusion of the common iliac artery: new approach to bleeding control during cesarean hysterectomy for placenta percreta. Am J Obstet Gynecol 2005;193(5):1756–8.

45. Greenberg JI, Suliman A, Iranpour P, et al. Prophylactic balloon occlusion of the internal iliac arteries to treat abnormal placentation: a cautionary case. Am J Obstet Gynecol 2007;197(5):470, e1–4.

46. Sewell MF, Rosenblum D, Ehrenberg H. Arterial embolus during common iliac balloon catheterization at cesarean hysterectomy. Obstet Gynecol 2006; 108(3 Pt 2):746–8.

47. Thon S, McLintic A, Wagner Y. Prophylactic endovascular placement of internal iliac occlusion balloon catheters in parturients with placenta accreta: a retrospective case series. Int J Obstet Anesth 2011;20(1):64–70.

48. Judlin P, Thiebaugeorges O. The ligation of hypogastric arteries is a safe alternative to balloon occlusion to treat abnormal placentation. Am J Obstet Gynecol 2008;199(3):e11 [author reply: e12–3].

49. Timmermans S, van Hof AC, Duvekot JJ. Conservative management of abnormally invasive placentation. Obstet Gynecol Surv 2007;62(8):529–39.

50. Sentilhes L, Ambroselli C, Kayem G, et al. Maternal outcome after conservative treatment of placenta accreta. Obstet Gynecol 2010;115(3):526–34.

Delivery After Prior Cesarean: Maternal Morbidity and Mortality

Yvonne W. Cheng, MD, MPH[a], Karen B. Eden, PhD[b],
Nicole Marshall, MD[c], Leonardo Pereira, MD[c],
Aaron B. Caughey, MD, PhD[d], Jeanne-Marie Guise, MD, MPH[e,f,*]

KEYWORDS

- VBAC • Pregnancy • Pregnancy complications
- Cesarean section • Evidence review

The dictum "Once a cesarean, always a cesarean" has largely permeated the obstetric practice for most of the twentieth century and today.[1] Although trial of labor after previous cesarean delivery (TOLAC) provides women who had a prior cesarean with an opportunity to achieve a vaginal birth after cesarean (VBAC), this was not

Financial disclosure: this work was funded by the Agency for Healthcare Research and Quality, contract no. HHSA 290-2007-10057-I, task order no. 4 for the Office of Medical Applications of Research at the National Institutes of Health.

[a] Division of Maternal-Fetal Medicine, Department of Obstetrics, Gynecology and Reproductive Sciences, University of California, San Francisco, 505 Parnassus Avenue, Box 0132, San Francisco, CA 94143, USA

[b] Department of Medical Informatics and Clinical Epidemiology, Oregon Evidence-based Practice Center, Oregon Health and Science University, Mail Code BICC, 3181 SW Sam Jackson Park Road, Portland, OR 97239, USA

[c] Division of Maternal-Fetal Medicine, Department of Obstetrics and Gynecology, Oregon Health & Science University, Mail Code L458, 3181 SW Sam Jackson Park Road, Portland, OR 97239, USA

[d] Department of Obstetrics and Gynecology, Oregon Health & Science University, Mail Code L466, 3181 SW Sam Jackson Park Road, Portland, OR 97239, USA

[e] Division of Maternal-Fetal Medicine, Departments of Obstetrics and Gynecology, Medical Informatics & Clinical Epidemiology, Public Health & Preventive Medicine, Oregon Evidence-based Practice Center, Oregon Health & Science University, Mail Code L466, 3181 SW Sam Jackson Park Road, Portland, OR 97239, USA

[f] Quality & Safety for Women's Services, Health Services & Outcomes Research, Oregon BIRCWH K12, Comparative Effectiveness K12 & KM1, Institute for Patient Centered Comparative Effectiveness, State Obstetric and Pediatric Research Collaborative (STORC), OHSU Center of Excellence in Women's Health, OHSU Hospital, Portland, OR 97239, USA

* Corresponding author. Division of Maternal-Fetal Medicine, Departments of Obstetrics and Gynecology, Medical Informatics & Clinical Epidemiology, Public Health & Preventive Medicine, Oregon Evidence-based Practice Center, Oregon Health & Science University, Mail Code L466, 3181 SW Sam Jackson Park Road, Portland, OR 97239.
E-mail address: guisej@ohsu.edu

Clin Perinatol 38 (2011) 297–309
doi:10.1016/j.clp.2011.03.012

considered a reasonable option until the 1970s to 1980s.[2–4] As the annual incidence of cesarean delivery increased from less than 5 per 100 live births during the 1970s to 23.5 per 100 live births in the United States in 1988,[5] the National Institute of Health (NIH) and the World Health Organization (WHO) held consensus conferences in the 1980s and concluded that cesarean delivery rates were too high and that VBAC was an acceptable approach for reducing cesarean delivery.[6,7] With this change in recommendations, the annual incidence of VBAC (defined as the number of VBACs per 100 women with a prior cesarean delivery per year) increased from 5/100 (5%) in 1985 to 28.3/100 (28.3%) in 1996.[8] At an individual level, successful VBAC is associated with a lower risk of maternal morbidity and fewer complications in future pregnancies; at a population level, VBAC is associated with an overall decrease in cesarean delivery.[9,10] However, neither elective repeat cesarean delivery (ERCD) nor TOLAC is without risks. With increasing number of TOLAC, there were also reports of uterine scar dehiscence or rupture and associated maternal and/or neonatal morbidity and mortality.[11–13] In the next decade, there was a steep decline in the frequency of VBAC down to an incidence of 8.5/100 (8.5%) in 2006,[14] likely caused by concern for perinatal morbidity and associated medical-legal liability.

The recent Practice Bulletin by the American College of Obstetricians and Gynecologists (ACOG) on Vaginal Birth After Previous Cesarean Delivery recommended that "most women with one previous cesarean delivery with a low transverse incision are candidates for and should be counseled about VBAC and offered TOLAC."[15] Despite this, the option of TOLAC is no longer available in one-third of hospitals[16] and clinicians are less inclined to offer TOLAC.[17] System-level changes, along with better identification of candidates of TOLAC, would likely be required to increase the VBAC rate.

This paper builds on a recent systematic evidence review conducted for the NIH Consensus Conference sponsored by the Agency for Healthcare Research and Quality (AHRQ) on VBAC[18] and 2 meta-analyses on prediction of VBAC[19] and associated perinatal outcomes.[20] It particularly emphasizes the information that clinicians and patients need to make decisions.

PRACTICE OF VBAC

The overall TOLAC among US studies was 58%, with a range of 28% to 70%.[18] For studies initiated after 1996, less than half of women (44%) had a TOLAC, compared with 62% of women in studies initiated before 1996.[18] Many factors, including site of delivery (rural vs urban), type of hospital (teaching vs community), history of prior vaginal delivery (including prior VBAC), and race/ethnicity (black and other minorities vs white), had been identified to modify TOLAC rates.[18,21–25] The incidence of VBAC among people who had TOLAC is approximately 74% in the United States.[18]

IDEAL CANDIDATES FOR VBAC

One of the greatest challenges in counseling and managing women with previous cesarean delivery regarding whether to undergo TOLAC versus ERCD is the inability to accurately identify women who have a high probability of VBAC and those who have increased risk of morbidity with TOLAC and thus may be better candidates for ERCD. Several factors have been identified to influence the likelihood of successful VBAC; these, in turn, can influence the decision to either undergo a trial of labor or proceed with elective repeat cesarean.

One of the strongest predictors of VBAC is previous vaginal delivery (Table 1). Studies consistently report that women with a history of vaginal delivery have a higher

| Table 1 |
| Factors associated with VBAC (↑, favorable factors; ↓, unfavorable factors) |

↑↑	Previous VBAC, previous vaginal deliveries
↑	Indication of prior cesarean as nonrecurring (eg, breech, fetal intolerance of labor)
↓	Hispanic compared with white; African American compared with white Increase in maternal age Increased maternal BMI Preexisting maternal medical disease Short interdelivery interval (<18 mo) Prolonged gestation >41 wk
↓↓	Indication of prior cesarean as recurring (eg, failure to progress, labor dystocia, or arrest of descent) Macrosomia (birthweight >4000 g)

Abbreviation: BMI, body mass index.

likelihood of VBAC than women who do not have prior vaginal deliveries. Although the probability of VBAC for women without history of vaginal delivery was 65%, women with prior vaginal delivery preceding cesarean had an 83% probability of achieving VBAC; for women with prior VBAC, the probability of subsequent successful VBAC was 94%.[26] A recent meta-analysis that examined predictors of VBAC similarly reported that prior vaginal delivery increases the odds of VBAC by more than threefold (odds ratio [OR] 3.41; 95% confidence interval [CI] 2.56–4.54).[19] More specifically, although having the experience of vaginal delivery is a favorable prognostic predictor of VBAC (a vaginal delivery preceding cesarean increased the odds of achieving VBAC [OR 1.60; 95% CI 1.22–2.09]), women who had prior VBAC had more than fourfold the odds of having VBAC again (OR 4.39; 95% CI 2.87–6.72).[19] Data from the National Institute of Child Health and Human Development Maternal-Fetal Medicine Units Network (MFMU) suggest that the number of prior VBACs remains positively correlated with increasing success of VBAC, such that, for women with 0, 1, 2, 3, and 4 or more prior VBACs, the likelihood of achieving VBAC in the current pregnancy was 63.3%, 87.6%, 90.9%, 90.6%, and 91.6%, respectively ($P<.001$).[27]

When the cesarean was performed for nonrecurrent indications, such as fetal malpresentation or breech, the probability of VBAC was approximately 75%.[18,19,28–30] One retrospective study reported that a previous cesarean delivery performed for malpresentation significantly increased the likelihood of VBAC (OR 7.4; 95% CI 2.8–19.2).[31] Another retrospective study also reported a similar association of VBAC for breech as the indication compared with nonbreech indications, although the estimated OR was smaller (OR 1.9; 95% CI 1.0–3.7).[32] These results were not pooled for meta-analysis because of differences in designation of reference comparisons but, overall, previous cesarean attributable to malpresentation as an indication was considered a favorable predictor of VBAC (see **Table 1**).[19] It was estimated that women with a previous cesarean for malpresentation carry a risk of repeat cesarean delivery that is similar to a nulliparous woman's risk of primary cesarean in labor: the estimated odds of repeat cesarean delivery is 0.95 (95% CI 0.7–1.30).[33]

Although previous cesarean for nonrecurring indications as discussed earlier is a favorable predictor of VBAC, it seems that the probability of achieving VBAC is lower if prior indication of cesarean was related to cephalopelvic disproportion (see **Table 1**).[18,19] More specifically, when failure to progress/active phase arrest, labor dystocia, arrest of descent, or cephalopelvic disproportion were the indications of previous cesarean, the likelihood of VBAC is about 54% (48%–60%).[18] The likelihood of VBAC is around 60% (49%–69%) if fetal intolerance of labor/fetal distress was the reason for prior cesarean.[18] Thus, compared with previous cesarean performed for nonrecurring indications (such as malpresentation/breech), women whose previous cesarean was performed for recurring indications had lower odds of achieving VBAC (adjusted OR [aOR] 0.42–0.8; 95% CI 0.3–0.6).[18,32,34,35]

Some obstetric factors (gestational age at delivery, birth weight) have been shown to modify the likelihood of VBAC (see **Table 1**). Infant birth weight is a strong predictor: as infant birth weight increases, the likelihood of VBAC decreases such that, for women whose infant weighed more than 4000 g, the probability of VBAC was reduced by 39% to 51% relative to that of women who had smaller infants.[35–38] A meta-analysis that examined 5 studies reported that women whose infant weighed more than 4000 g had nearly half the likelihood of VBAC (OR 0.55; 95% CI 0.49–0.61).[19] However, infant birth weight is not known before delivery, and estimating fetal weight in the third trimester is notoriously challenging and inaccurate.[39,40] Several studies also examined gestational age as a predictor of VBAC, but they varied in study design and thus pooled estimates of effect cannot be generated, although the overall trend seems to be that, as gestational age increases, the likelihood of VBAC is decreased, particularly when the pregnancy progresses beyond 41 weeks' gestation.[19]

Several maternal demographic factors have been examined for their potential to improve the clinician's ability to predict VBAC (see **Table 1**). Of the many demographic predictors, the strongest and most consistent seems to be race/ethnicity.[19] Three cohort studies report that, compared with non-Hispanic white women, Hispanic women and African American women had a lower likelihood of achieving a VBAC: a reduction of 29% to 50% for Hispanic women and 20% to 52% for African Americans.[34,41,42] When these studies were examined in a meta-analysis, Hispanic women had a significantly reduced odds of VBAC (pooled OR 0.59; 95% CI 0.50–0.71) as did African American women (pooled OR 0.62; 95% CI 0.48–0.80) compared with white women.[19] Although nonwhite women were more likely to undergo a TOLAC, they were less likely to achieve VBAC; the reasons for this remain unclear.[25] Studies that examined the association between maternal age and VBAC report an inverse relationship: older women are less likely to have a VBAC (see **Table 1**). Compared with women aged 40 years or younger, women older than 40 years had nearly half the likelihood of VBAC in a meta-analysis (OR 0.53; 95% CI 0.32–0.86).[19] When age was examined as a continuous variable, for every 5-year incremental increase in maternal age, the odds of VBAC also decreased (OR 0.83; 95% CI 0.79–0.87).[19] When maternal age was examined as a risk factor for needing emergency cesarean in the setting of TOLAC, a positive association was again seen (OR 1.22 per incremental 5-year increase in age; 95% CI 1.16–1.28).[43]

Other maternal characteristics that can modify the likelihood of VBAC are maternal weight and presence of medical conditions (see **Table 1**). Increasing maternal body mass index (BMI) at first prenatal visit or at delivery decreases the probability of VBAC.[34,37] Each unit increase in BMI at first prenatal visit decreases the likelihood of VBAC (OR 0.94; 95% CI 0.93–0.95).[34] Compared with nonobese women (BMI<30 kg/m^2), women with a BMI greater than or equal to 30 kg/m^2 at delivery have much lower odds of VBAC (OR 0.55; 95% CI 0.51–60).[37] Because many medical conditions complicating pregnancy are associated with increased risk of cesarean delivery, 3 large cohort studies reported that women with medical diseases were less likely to have VBAC, by 17% to 58%, with the following aORs: chronic hypertension (OR 0.70; 95% CI 0.56–0.86); diabetes/gestational diabetes (OR 0.42; 95% CI 0.28–0.62); and presence of any hypertension, diabetes, asthma, seizures, renal disease, thyroid disease, or collagen vascular disease (OR 0.83; 95% CI 071–0.91).[35,37,42]

There is considerable interest in whether the number of prior cesareans affects the likelihood of VBAC (see **Table 1**). Because most studies of TOLAC/VBAC focus on women with 1 prior cesarean delivery, data on TOLAC in women with more than 1 previous cesarean delivery are less clear. Two large, multicenter cohort studies report that the probability of achieving successful VBAC appears to be similar for women with 1 prior cesarean (75.5%) or more than 1 cesarean delivery (74.6%), although 1 study reported higher risks of uterine rupture whereas the other did not.[44,45] Thus, the ACOG practice bulletin on VBAC stated that, "it is reasonable to consider women with 2 previous low transverse cesarean deliveries to be candidates for TOLAC, and to counsel them based on the combination of other factors that affect their probability of achieving a successful VBAC."[15] Data on the risks and outcomes of women undergoing TOLAC with 3 or more previous cesarean deliveries are scant. One multicenter cohort study did not observe any cases of composite maternal morbidity and noted a similar probability of achieving VBAC (79.8%) for women with 3 or more previous cesareans as for women with 1 prior cesarean delivery (75.5%; aOR 1.4; 95% CI 0.81–2.41).[46]

CONSIDERATIONS FOR ANTEPARTUM AND INTRAPARTUM MANAGEMENT OF WOMEN WITH PRIOR CESAREAN
Induction/Augmentation of Labor and VBAC

Induction of labor (IOL) for maternal or fetal indications is increasingly common in obstetric practice and has increased from 9.5% in 1990 to 22.8% in 2007 in the United States[47] Although TOLAC remains an option in women for whom induction of labor is indicated, labor induction and augmentation is associated with a decreased likelihood of VBAC (OR 0.56; 95% CI 0.38–0.83.[18,19] Most studies on this topic examined the use of prostaglandin E_2 (PGE_2) as the cervical ripening agent: the pooled estimates of VBAC rate in women with previous cesarean who received PGE_2 for IOL was approximately 63% (95% CI 58%–69%).[18] Data on misoprostol or mifepristone as IOL agents are more limited; the pooled estimates of VBAC rate range between 61% and 69%.[18] Although oxytocin can be used alone for the purpose of induction or for augmentation of labor, studies that examined use of oxytocin as an induction agent estimated the probability of VBAC to be 62% (95% CI 53%–70%); as an augmentation agent, oxytocin is similarly associated with decreased probability of VBAC (68%; 95% CI 64%–72%).[18] The pooled estimates from a meta-analysis report that women whose labor required oxytocin augmentation had nearly half the likelihood of VBAC compared with those who did not (OR 0.52; 95% CI 0.33–0.82).[19]

Cervical Status at Admission and VBAC

The likelihood of VBAC may be modified by intrapartum conditions such as cervical status and labor progression. Some studies have reported that women admitted with a more favorable cervical status (eg, cervical dilation >4 cm, advanced effacement) in spontaneous labor have a twofold increase in the likelihood of VBAC compared with those with unfavorable cervix (OR 2.2–2.6; 95% CI 1.7–2.8).[19,37,48] When As a continuous variable, each centimeter in cervical dilatation at admission is associated with increased odds of VBAC (OR 1.89; 95% CI 1.13–3.22).[49] More than 75% effacement of the cervix (compared with 25% effacement) at admission also increases the likelihood of VBAC (OR 2.72; 95% CI 2.00–3.71).[48]

OUTCOMES OF TRIAL OF LABOR VERSUS ERCD FOR INDEX PREGNANCY

Because a successful VBAC cannot be guaranteed, and because risks versus benefits may be disproportionately associated with a failed trial of labor after cesarean (in which a woman undergoes a repeat cesarean delivery after a trial of labor) compared with an elective repeat cesarean or a successful VBAC, the appropriate statistical comparison for both research and patient counseling regarding mode of delivery for women with a previous cesarean is by intention to deliver: TOLAC versus ERCD.[18] This article focuses on the risks of morbidity associated with TOLAC and those associated with ERCD.

Maternal Death

Despite improvement in medical technology and care, maternal mortality increased from 7 to 9 per 100,000 in the 1980s and 1990s to 12 to 15 per 100,000 since 2003.[50,51] Although the absolute risk of maternal death remains low, a meta-analysis found that maternal mortality is higher for ERCD, at 13.4 per 100,000 (95% CI 4.3–41.6 per 100,000 ERCD) compared with 3.8 per 100,000 TOLAC (95% CI 0.9–15.5 per 100,000 TOLAC).[18,20] One study examined whether hospitals with low delivery volumes (defined as fewer than 500 deliveries per year) were associated with increased odds of maternal mortality with TOLAC and did not observe a statistical significance because of the small number of maternal deaths.[52]

Uterine Rupture

Uterine rupture is potentially life threatening and catastrophic for the expecting mother and her fetus(es), and it is the outcome associated with TOLAC that most significantly increases the risk of perinatal morbidity and mortality.[9,18] Among studies that examined uterine rupture for both TOLAC and ERCD groups, the overall incidence of uterine rupture was 0.30% (95% CI 0.23%–0.40%); however, 96% of ruptures occurred in women who had TOLAC.[18] Thus, despite the absolute risk of uterine rupture remaining low, the risk of uterine rupture is higher for women undergoing TOLAC than ERCD (Table 2). In addition, the occurrence of uterine rupture was higher for studies limited to term pregnancies compared with studies that included women of any gestational age at delivery (0.78% vs 0.32%, respectively; $P = .03$).[18] When the direction of previous uterine incision was examined as a risk factor for uterine rupture, one multi-center cohort study reported that women with a low, transverse cesarean delivery or an unknown scar have the lowest risk of rupture (0.63%–0.75%).[18,53]

Another factor that may modify the risk of uterine rupture is IOL. More specifically, the risk of uterine rupture among women who had induction was lowest with oxytocin (1.1%), followed by PGE_2 (2%), and highest with misoprostol (6%); however, these risk estimations may be imprecise given the consistency in study design and methodology, so these results should be interpreted with caution.[18] In particular, the method of induction is likely associated with the cervical status as well as the duration of

Table 2 Maternal outcomes associated with TOLAC versus ERCD			
	Favors TOLAC	Favors ERCD	No Difference
Maternal death	✔	—	—
Uterine rupture	—	✔	—
Hysterectomy	—	—	✔
Hemorrhage and transfusion	—	—	✔
Infection	—	—	✔
Surgical injury	—	—	✔

induction, which may confound the strength of the associations reported in many studies. Individual factors associated with uterine rupture included increasing maternal age, prior vaginal delivery or VBAC, increased number of previous cesarean deliveries, increased gestational age at delivery, shorter interpregnancy interval, induction/augmentation of labor, epidural anesthesia, and having a single-layer uterine closure on previous cesarean.[18]

Although the presence of risk factors may help identify women at higher risk of uterine rupture, the diagnosis of rupture can be challenging because there is no single sign that reliably indicates the occurrence of rupture. Fetal heart rate tracing abnormalities, especially fetal bradycardia (reported in 33%–100% of uterine ruptures), are the most commonly observed signs of uterine rupture.[3,54–56] Others include maternal vaginal bleeding, pain, and abnormal uterine contraction patterns.[48]

Hysterectomy

Among the 8 studies that examined the risk of hysterectomy among women with previous cesarean, the summary incidence was 0.28% for women who had ERCD (95% CI 0.12%–0.67%) and 0.17% for women who had a trial of labor (95% CI 0.12%–0.26%), which were not statistically significantly different (see **Table 2**).[18] Among term pregnancies, the incidence of hysterectomy among women who had TOLAC and ERCD were similar (0.14% vs 0.16%, respectively; $P = .67$). When the risk of hysterectomy was compared among women who had TOLAC after 1 cesarean, TOLAC after 2 or more cesareans, and ERCD, the incidence of hysterectomy was lowest among women with TOLAC after 1 cesarean delivery (0.2%), whereas it was 0.4% among women who had ERCD, and highest (0.6%) among women who had TOLAC after multiple previous cesareans.[36]

Hemorrhage and Transfusion

Studies report increased rates of hemorrhage associated with ERCD (0.3%–29%) compared with TOLAC, but none found a statistically significant difference between the 2 groups (see **Table 2**).[18] Inconsistent definitions of hemorrhage used by various studies probably contributed to the wide range of hemorrhage rates reported. In addition, physicians' estimation of blood loss has been known to be imprecise and this adds to the challenge of studying this topic.[18] Because these studies did not use similar definitions to diagnose hemorrhage, these data were not combined to provide pooled estimates.

The difference in pooled incidences of transfusion among women who had TOLAC (0.9%) and women who had ERCD (1.2%) was not statistically significant (see **Table 2**).[18] However, when data were limited to only term pregnancies, the risk of transfusion was higher for TOLAC (0.7%; 95% CI 0.2%–2.2%) than for ERCD (0.5%; 95% CI 0.2%–1.3%), with a relative risk (RR) that is higher for TOLAC (RR 1.30; 95% CI 1.15 to 1.4).[18] When the risk of transfusion was stratified among women who had ERCD and women who had indicated repeat cesarean (IRCD) with or without labor, women who had IRCD without labor had a higher risk of transfusion, suggesting that maternal comorbid conditions contribute to the risk of transfusion.[53]

Infection

There was no significant difference in the overall infection risk between women who had TOLAC and women who had ERCD (see **Table 2**).[18] When infection was further stratified by type (endometritis, chorioamnionitis, wound infection, and fever), a higher risk of endometritis was seen in women who had TOLAC (0.8%–30%) than those who had ERCD (1.2%–18%).[18] There was a significant increase in the rate of endometritis with increasing BMI such that, in morbidly obese women (BMI >40 kg/m²), TOLAC is associated with more than twice the odds of endometritis than ERCD (aOR 2.4; 95% CI 1.7–3.5).[57] Similarly, a higher incidence of chorioamnionitis was seen in women who had TOLAC compared with those who had ERCD.[58,59] There was no statistically significant difference in the risk of wound infection in TOLAC compared with ERCD.[18] The pooled incidence of febrile morbidity was 6.5% (95% CI 4.4%–9.3%) for women who had TOLAC and 7.2% (2.5%–18.9%) for women who had ERCD; the relative risk of fever for TOLAC was significantly lower than ERCD (RR 0.63; 95% CI 0.43–0.91).[18] When the association of fever was further evaluated by outcomes of TOLAC, women who had either cesarean after a trial of labor or ERCD had higher risk compared with those who had successful VBAC, thus suggesting surgery as a risk factor for febrile morbidity.[18,59,60]

Surgical Injury

Surgical injury is a rare complication during delivery. Secondary data analyses from a multicentered large cohort study suggest that the risk of surgical injury between TOLAC and ERCD was not statistically significantly different (see **Table 2**).[18,46,53,57,61]

CONSIDERATIONS FOR FUTURE PREGNANCIES AND THE IMPACT OF MULTIPLE CESAREANS

Women who choose an ERCD or those who have an unsuccessful TOLAC will likely require cesarean delivery for all future pregnancies, making it important to understand the risks, including hysterectomy and placental abnormalities, associated with multiple prior cesareans.

Hysterectomy

Hysterectomy rates increased with each additional cesarean in all studies.[4,13,16,17,19,20,22] The OR for hysterectomy increased with the number of prior cesareans, from 0.7 to 2.14 with 1 prior cesarean, 1.4 to 7.9 with 1 or more prior cesareans, and to 3.8 to 18.6 with 2 or more prior cesareans. The association between increased risk of hemorrhage, blood transfusion, surgical injury, and adhesions with increasing number of cesarean deliveries was consistently reported in all studies.[18,20] Increasing number of cesarean deliveries was not associated with a change in perioperative infection or wound complications.

Placenta Previa

Prior cesarean was a statistically significant risk factor for placenta previa compared with prior normal spontaneous vaginal delivery (NSVD; OR 1.48–3.95).[18] The pooled analysis estimated the absolute risk of previa associated with any number of cesareans as 12 per 1000 (95% CI 8, 15 per 1000; P<.001).[20] The incidence with each additional prior cesarean delivery increased from 10 per 1000 with 1 prior cesarean delivery (95% CI 6, 13 per 1000) to 28 per 1000 (95% CI 18, 37 per 1000) with 3 or more cesarean deliveries. Women with no prior cesarean delivery and previa required hysterectomy in 0.7% to 4% of cases compared with 50% to 67% in women with 3 or more prior cesarean deliveries.[34,62–64]

Placenta Accreta

The incidence of placenta accreta increased with increasing number of cesarean deliveries. The increased incidence did not reach statistical significance until women had at least 2 prior cesarean deliveries compared with no prior cesarean delivery

(OR 8.6–29.8).[18] Women with 1 prior cesarean delivery had a rate of accreta of 0.3% to 0.6%. In comparison with women without prior cesarean delivery, the OR for accreta with 1 prior cesarean delivery was 1.3 to 2.16, which was not statistically significant. The incidence of accreta continued to increase with increasing prior cesarean delivery up to 6.74% for women with 5 or more prior cesarean delivery compared with no prior cesarean delivery, with an OR of 29.8.[18]

Two studies noted a statistically significant increase in accreta in women with previa and prior cesarean delivery.[3,4] As the number of prior cesarean delivery increased, the presence of placenta previa increased the likelihood of placenta accreta from 3.3% to 4% in women undergoing their first cesarean delivery to 50% to 67% in women with 4 or more prior cesarean delivery. The risk of hysterectomy in women with accreta and prior cesarean delivery was not reported separately, but 2 studies found that accreta was a significant risk factor for hysterectomy (OR 43–99.5; 95% CI 19.0, ∞).[13,16]

Each additional cesarean is associated with increased maternal morbidity in a dose-response fashion, especially for women with 3 or more prior cesareans, who are at statistically significant increased risk of previa, accreta, and hysterectomy.

SHARED DECISION MAKING AND COUNSELING

For most of the twentieth century, "Once a cesarean, always a cesarean" was the standard obstetric practice. Although TOLAC is deemed an appropriate option in women with previous cesarean delivery, assessment of individual risks and the likelihood of successful VBAC are important in determining who may be appropriate candidates for TOLAC. Much effort has been put forth to improve the identification of prognostic factors associated VBAC and to develop normograms for predicting VBAC and associated morbidity.[31,34,49,65] In addition, patient involvement in the decision-making process and counseling of TOLAC/VBAC has been associated with increased choice of TOLAC as well as increased patient satisfaction. Early timing of counseling is likely to be important because nearly half of the women with prior cesarean make decisions about future TOLAC before becoming pregnant again.[19]

Ideally, good candidates for planned TOLAC are women in whom the balance between risks (desirably as low as possible) and success (as high as possible) is acceptable both to the patient and the clinician. However, this is often an individual decision, and what is considered acceptable for 1 patient may be different for another. Thus, counseling of women with previous cesarean delivery who are considering their delivery options involves personalized information. The key in facilitating a woman's decision with respect to undergoing a TOLAC is proper counseling regarding her chances of success, a uterine rupture, and injury to herself or fetus if she experiences a uterine rupture.

Informed consent today for any woman who desires a TOLAC must address 4 specific questions: (1) what is her chance of having a successful VBAC? (2) What is the risk that she will have a uterine rupture if she does attempt a VBAC? (3) What is the chance of harm or death to her baby if the uterus ruptures? (4) What are the risks of undergoing a repeat cesarean delivery? In addition, future fertility/family plans present as a key factor that should be considered because multiple cesareans increase a woman's risk for future pregnancy complications. In particular, the risk of placenta previa, accreta, and hysterectomy increases in a dose-response fashion with increasing number of cesarean deliveries, so clinicians should elucidate future pregnancy/family plans and incorporate such in the decision-making process with the patient.

SUMMARY

The annual incidence of cesarean delivery in the United States continues to increase such that today, nearly 1 in 3 pregnant women undergo cesarean.[48] This trend is contrary to the national goal of decreasing cesarean delivery in low-risk women.[66,67] Although there are many potential causes, the decline in VBACs contributes to the continual increase in cesarean deliveries. Prior cesarean delivery is the most common indication for cesarean and accounts for more than one-third of all cesareans. As the most common inpatient surgical procedure performed in the United States, cesarean delivery also accounts for nearly half of the childbirth-related expenses of hospitalization, at $7.8 billion annually.[18] Thus, the appropriate use and safety of cesarean and VBAC are of concern not only at the individual patient and clinician level but they also have far-reaching public health and policy implications at the national level. Although TOLAC/VBAC is a reasonable and safe option for most women with prior cesarean delivery, careful consideration of risks/benefits and assessment of individual factors is vital in this decision-making process.

REFERENCES

1. Cragin EB. Conservatism in obstetrics. NY Med J 1916;104:1–3.
2. Lavin JP, Stephens RJ, Miodovnik M, et al. Vaginal delivery in patients with a prior cesarean section. Obstet Gynecol 1982;59:135–48.
3. Flamm BL, Newman LA, Thomas SJ, et al. Vaginal birth after cesarean delivery: results of a 5-year multicenter collaborative study. Obstet Gynecol 1990;76:750–4.
4. Miller DA, Diaz FG, Paul RH. Vaginal birth after cesarean: a 10-year experience. Obstet Gynecol 1994;84:255–8.
5. Centers for Disease Control and Prevention (CDC). Rates of cesarean delivery—United States 1991. MMWR Morb Mortal Wkly Rep 1993;42:285–9.
6. Cesarean Childbirth: report of a Consensus Development Conference. Sponsored by the NICHD in conjunction with the National Center for Health Care Technology and assisted by the Office for Medical Applications of Research. Washington, DC: NIH Publication; 1981. p. 82–2067.
7. Appropriate technology for birth. Lancet 1985;2:436–7.
8. Menacker F, Declercq E, Macdorman MF. Cesarean delivery: background, trends, and epidemiology. Semin Perinatol 2006;30:235–41.
9. American College of Obstetricians and Gynecologists. Practice Bulletin: Clinical management guidelines for obstetrician-gynecologists. Vaginal birth after previous cesarean delivery. Obstet Gynecol 2010;116:450–63.
10. Curtin SC. Rates of cesarean birth and vaginal birth after previous cesarean, 1991–95. Mon Vital Stat Rep 1997;45(11 Suppl 3):1–12.
11. Sachs BP, Kobelin C, Castro MA, et al. The risks of lowering the cesarean-delivery rate. N Engl J Med 1999;340:54–7.
12. Phelan JP. VBAC: time to reconsider? OBG Management 1996;8:64–8.
13. Caughey AB, Shipp TD, Repke JT, et al. Rate of uterine rupture during a trial of labor in women with one or two prior cesarean deliveries. Am J Obstet Gynecol 1999;181:872–6.
14. Martin JA, Hamilton EB, Sutton PD, et al. Births: final data for 2006. Natl Vital Stat Rep 2009;57:1–104.
15. The American College of Obstetricians and Gynecologists Practice Bulletin—Clinical Guidelines for Obstetrician-Gynecologists. Vaginal birth after previous cesarean delivery. No 115, August 2010 (replaces Practice Bulletin No 54, July 2004 and Committee Opinion No 342, August 2006). Obstet Gynecol 2010;116:450–63.

16. National Institutes of Health. NIH Consensus Development Conference: vaginal birth after cesarean: new insights. Consensus Development Conference statement. Bethesda (MD): NIH; 2010. Available at: http://consensus.nih.gov/2010/images/vbac/vbac_statement.pdf. Accessed November 9, 2010.

17. Angelini DJ, Greenwald L. Closed claims analysis of 65 medical malpractice cases involving nurse-midwives. J Midwifery Womens Health 2005;50:454–60.

18. Guise JM, Eden K, Emeis C, et al. Vaginal birth after cesarean: new insights. Evidence Report/Technology Assessment No. 191 (Prepared by the Oregon Health & Science University Evidence-based Practice Center under contract no. 290-2008-10057-I). AHRQ Publication No. 10-E003. Rockville (MD): Agency for Healthcare Research and Quality; 2010.

19. Eden KB, McDonagh M, Denman MA, et al. New insights on vaginal birth after cesarean: can it be predicted? Obstet Gynecol 2010;116:967–81.

20. Guise JM, Denman MA, Emeis C, et al. Vaginal birth after cesarean: new insights on maternal and neonatal outcomes. Obstet Gynecol 2010;115:1267–78.

21. McMahon MJ, Luther ER, Bowes WA Jr, et al. Comparison of a trial of labor with an elective second cesarean section. N Engl J Med 1996;335:689–95.

22. Cameron CA, Roberts CL, Peat B. Predictors of labor and vaginal birth after cesarean section. Int J Gynaecol Obstet 2004;85:267–9.

23. Hueston WJ, Rudy M. Factors predicting elective repeat cesarean delivery. Obstet Gynecol 1994;83:741–4.

24. Pang MW, Law LW, Leung TY, et al. Sociodemographic factors and pregnancy events associated with women who declined vaginal birth after cesarean section. Eur J Obstet Gynecol Reprod Biol 2009;143:24–8.

25. Selo-Ojeme D, Abulhassan N, Mandal R, et al. Preferred and actual delivery mode after cesarean in London, UK. Int J Gynaecol Obstet 2008;102:156–9.

26. Elkousy MA, Sammel M, Stevens E, et al. The effect of birthweight on vaginal birth after cesarean delivery success rates. Am J Obstet Gynecol 2003;188:824–30.

27. Mercer BM, Gilbert S, Landon MB, et al. Labor outcomes with increasing number of prior vaginal births after cesarean delivery. Obstet Gynecol 2008;111:285–91.

28. Van Gelderen CJ, England MJ, Naylor GA, et al. Labour in patients with a cesarean section scar. The place of oxytocin augmentation. S Afr Med J 1998;70:529–32.

29. Horenstein JM, Eglinston GS, Tahilramaney MP, et al. Oxytocin use during a trial of labor in patients with previous cesarean section. J Reprod Med 1984;29:26–30.

30. Flamm BL, Goings JR, Fuelberth NJ, et al. Oxytocin during labor after previous cesarean section: results of a multicenter study. Obstet Gynecol 1987;70:709–12.

31. Gonen R, Tamir A, Degani S, et al. Variables associated with successful vaginal birth after one cesarean section: a proposed vaginal birth after cesarean section score. Am J Perinatol 2004;21:447–53.

32. Weinstein D, Benshushan A, Tanos V, et al. Predictive score for vaginal delivery after cesarean section. Am J Obstet Gynecol 1996;174:192–8.

33. Shipp TD, Zelop CM, Repke JT, et al. Labor after previous cesarean: influence of prior indication and parity. Obstet Gynecol 2000;95:913–6.

34. Grobman WA, Lai Y, Landon MB, et al. Development of a nomogram for prediction of vaginal birth after cesarean delivery. Obstet Gynecol 2007;109:806–12.

35. Gyamfi C, Juhasz G, Gyamfi P, et al. Increased success of trial of labor after previous vaginal birth after cesarean. Obstet Gynecol 2004;104:715–9.

36. Landon MB, Spong CY, Thom E, et al. Risk of uterine rupture with a trial of labor in women with multiple and single prior cesarean delivery. Obstet Gynecol 2006;108:12–20.

37. Landon MB, Leindecker S, Spong CY, et al. The MFMU Cesarean Registry: factors affecting the success of trial of labor after previous cesarean delivery. Am J Obstet Gynecol 2005;193:1016–23.

38. Zelop CM, Shipp TD, Cohen A, et al. Trial of labor after 40 weeks' gestation in women with prior cesarean. Obstet Gynecol 2001;97:391–3.

39. Chauhan SP, Cowan BD, Magann EF, et al. Intrapartum detection of a macrosomic fetus: clinical versus 8 sonographic models. Aust N Z J Obstet Gynaecol 1995; 35:266–70.

40. Hiratal GI, Medearis AL, Horenstein J, et al. Ultrasonographic estimation of fetal weight in the clinically macrosomic fetus. Am J Obstet Gynecol 1990;162:238–42.

41. King DE, Lahiri K. Socioeconomic factors and the odds of vaginal birth after cesarean delivery. JAMA 1994;272:524–9.

42. Srinivas SK, Stamilio DM, Stevens EJ, et al. Predicting failure of a vaginal birth attempt after cesarean delivery. Obstet Gynecol 2007;109:800–5.

43. Smith GC, White IR, Pell JP, et al. Predicting cesarean section and uterine rupture among women attempting vaginal birth after prior cesarean section. PLoS Med 2005;2:e252.

44. Macones GA, Cahill A, Pare E, et al. Obstetric outcomes in women with two prior cesarean deliveries: is vaginal birth after cesarean delivery a viable option? Am J Obstet Gynecol 2005;192:1223–8.

45. Asakura H, Myers SA. More than one previous cesarean delivery: a 5-year experience with 435 patients. Obstet Gynecol 1995;95:924–9.

46. Cahill AG, Tuuli M, Odibo AO, et al. Vaginal birth after cesarean for women with three or more prior cesareans: assessing safety and success. BJOG 2010;117: 422–7.

47. Martin JA, Hamilton BE, Sutton PD, et al. Birth: final data for 2007. Natl Vital Stat Rep 2010;58:1–125.

48. Flamm BL, Geiger AM. Vaginal birth after cesarean delivery: an admission scoring system. Obstet Gynecol 1997;90:907–10.

49. Macones GA, Hausman N, Edelstein R, et al. Predicting outcomes of trials of labor in women attempting vaginal birth after cesarean delivery: a comparison of multivariate methods with neural networks. Am J Obstet Gynecol 2001;194: 409–13.

50. Hoyert DL. Maternal mortality and related concepts. Vital Health Stat 2007;33: 1–13.

51. Kung HC, Hoyert DL, Xu J, et al. Death: final data for 2005. Natl Vital Stat Rep 2008;56:1–120.

52. Wen SW, Rusen ID, Walker M, et al. Maternal Health Study Group, Canadian Perinatal Surveillance System. Comparison of maternal mortality and morbidity between trial of labor and elective cesarean section among women with previous cesarean delivery. Am J Obstet Gynecol 2004;191:1263–9.

53. Spong CY, Landon MB, Gilbert S, et al. National Institute of Child Health and Human Development (NICHD) Maternal-Fetal Medicine Units (MFMU) Network. Risk of uterine rupture and adverse perinatal outcome at term after cesarean delivery. Obstet Gynecol 2007;110:801–7.

54. Guise JM, McDonagh MS, Hashima J, et al. Vaginal birth after cesarean (VBAC). Evid Rep Technol Assess (Summ) 2003;(71):1–8.

55. Cowan RK, Kinch RA, Ellis B, et al. Trial of labor following cesarean delivery. Obstet Gynecol 1994;83:933–6.

56. Flamm BL, Lim OW, Jones C, et al. Vaginal birth after cesarean section: results of a multicenter study. Am J Obstet Gynecol 1998;158:1079–84.

57. Hibbard JU, Gilbert S, Landon MB, et al. Trial of labor or repeat cesarean delivery in women with morbid obesity and previous cesarean delivery. Obstet Gynecol 2006;108:125–33.
58. Kugler E, Shoham-Vardi I, Burstein E, et al. The safety of a trial of labor after cesarean section in a grandmultiparous population. Arch Gynecol Obstet 2008; 277:339–44.
59. Dumwald C, Mercer B. Vaginal birth after cesarean delivery: predicting success, risks of failure. J Matern Fetal Neonatal Med 2004;15:388–93.
60. Eglinton GS, Phelan JP, Yeh S, et al. Outcome of a trial of labor after prior cesarean delivery. J Reprod Med 1984;29:3–8.
61. Silver RM, Landon MB, Rouse DJ, et al. Maternal morbidity associated with multiple repeat cesarean deliveries. Obstet Gynecol 2006;107:1226–32.
62. Zelop CM, Harlow BL, Frigoletto FD Jr, et al. Emergency peripartum hysterectomy. Am J Obstet Gynecol 1993;168:1443–8.
63. Juntunen K, Makarainen L, Kirkinen P. Outcome after a high number (4–10) of repeat cesarean sections. BJOG 2004;111:561–3.
64. Lynch CM, Kearney R, Turner MJ. Maternal morbidity after elective repeat cesarean section after two or more previous procedures. Eur J Obstet Gynecol Reprod Biol 2003;106:10–3.
65. Grobman WA, Lai Y, Landon MB, et al. Can a prediction model for vaginal birth after cesarean also predict the probability of morbidity related to a trial of labor? Am J Obstet Gynecol 2009;200:56,e1–6.
66. Healthy People 2010. Maternal, infant, and child health. Department of Health and Human Services. Available at: http://www.healthypeople.gov/2010/Data/midcourse/html/focusareas/FA16ProgressHP.htm. Accessed November 9, 2010.
67. Healthy People 2020. Maternal, infant, and child health. Department of Health and Human Services. Available at: http://www.healthypeople.gov/HP2020/Objectives/ViewObjective.aspx?Id=161&TopicArea=Maternal%2c+Infant+and+Child+Health&Objective=MICH+HP2020%e2%80%936&TopicAreaId=32. Accessed November 9, 2010.

Fetal and Neonatal Morbidity and Mortality Following Delivery After Previous Cesarean

Mitzi Donabel A. Go, MD[a], Cathy Emeis, PhD[b],
Jeanne-Marie Guise, MD, MPH[c,d,e], Robert L. Schelonka, MD[a,*]

KEYWORDS

- VBAC • Pregnancy • Pregnancy complications
- Cesarean section • Evidence review

The effective and safe use of cesarean section for delivery has been a focus of national attention and concern for decades. This national introspection is justified, as today nearly one-third of all infants will be born by cesarean delivery, making it the most commonly performed major surgical procedure in the United States.[1–3] There has been more than a sevenfold increase in cesarean deliveries in the United States, from 4.5% in 1965 to 32.5% in 2008.[1,2] The increase in the rate of cesarean is complex, perpetuated by the dictum "once a cesarean, always a cesarean,"[3] but also a result of changes in obstetric practices, including the introduction of electronic

Financial Disclosure: This work was funded by the Agency for Healthcare Research and Quality, Contract No. HHSA 290-2007-10057-I, Task order No. 4 for the Office of Medical Applications of Research at the National Institutes of Health.

[a] Division of Neonatology, Department of Pediatrics, Oregon Health & Science University, Mail code CDRCP, 707 Southwest Gaines Street, Portland, OR 97239-2998, USA
[b] Nurse-Midwifery Program, School of Nursing, Oregon Health & Science University, Mail code SN-5S, 3455 SW US Veterans Hospital Road, Portland, OR 97239, USA
[c] Division of Maternal-Fetal Medicine, Department of Obstetrics and Gynecology, Oregon Evidence-based Practice Center, Oregon Health & Science University, Mail code L466, 3181 SW Sam Jackson Park Road, Portland, OR 97239, USA
[d] Department of Medical Informatics and Clinical Epidemiology, Oregon Evidence-based Practice Center, Oregon Health & Science University, Mail code L466, 3181 SW Sam Jackson Park Road, Portland, OR 97239, USA
[e] Department of Public Health and Preventive Medicine, Oregon Evidence-based Practice Center, Oregon Health & Science University, Mail code L466, 3181 SW Sam Jackson Park Road, Portland, OR 97239, USA
* Corresponding author.
E-mail address: schelonk@ohsu.edu

Clin Perinatol 38 (2011) 311–319
doi:10.1016/j.clp.2011.03.001
0095-5108/11/$ – see front matter © 2011 Elsevier Inc. All rights reserved.

fetal monitoring, increasing numbers of multiple-gestation pregnancies, and the decrease in vaginal breech and forceps-assisted deliveries.[4] Vaginal birth after caesarean (VBAC) emerged from the 1980 National Institutes of Health (NIH) Consensus Conference on Cesarean Childbirth as a mechanism to safely reduce this rate.[5] However, since 1996, there has been a downward trend in trial of labor after cesarean (TOLAC) rates.[6] Most women who have TOLAC will have a VBAC, and they and their infants will be healthy; however, a minority of women will suffer serious adverse consequences of both TOLAC and elective repeat cesarean delivery (ERCD).

Although both failed TOL and cesarean delivery are associated with maternal risks, trends of increasing cesarean deliveries are driven at least in part by fears of the perceived risk of VBAC to the fetus. The most concerning complication of TOLAC is maternal uterine rupture, which has been associated with fetal demise or substantial neonatal morbidity. It has been difficult to ascertain comparative risks and benefits of VBAC and ERCD to the fetus and neonate.[4] This article examines data from a recent systematic evidence review on term deliveries conducted for the NIH Consensus Conference sponsored by the Agency for Healthcare Research and Quality (AHRQ) on VBAC,[6] from a meta-analysis of associated perinatal outcomes,[7] and subsequent publications that meet the same stringent quality review standards as the evidence reviews. We present a summary of fetal and neonatal outcomes (**Table 1**) emphasizing information that clinicians and patients need to make decisions regarding mode of delivery after prior cesarean and look for areas where future studies may provide important insights.

MORTALITY

The ability to provide accurate estimates of risk of death to the fetus in women contemplating a TOLAC versus ERCD is as important as providing patients with estimates of the risk of maternal death. Understanding the risk of death to the fetus in pregnancy and birth, regardless of mode of delivery, requires examining perinatal mortality and its subsets of fetal and neonatal mortality.

Perinatal mortality, which includes fetal and neonatal death up to 28 days,[8] is of paramount concern when considering the safety of VBAC and ERCD. Five cohort

Table 1 Directionality of risk for neonatal outcomes associated with TOLAC	
	TOLAC Associated Risk[a]
Mortality	
Perinatal	↑
Neonatal	↑
Resuscitation	
Mild/Moderate	↓
BMV	↑
Apgar, 5 minute	↔
Neonatal admission	?
Respiratory conditions	
Transient tachypnea	↔
Hypoxic ischemic encephalopathy	?

Abbreviations: BMV, bag-and-mask ventilation; TOLAC, trial of labor after cesarean.
[a] See text for details.

studies[8–12] met study criteria established in the NIH/AHRQ systematic evidence review.[7] All 5 studies focused exclusively on women delivering at term, thereby reducing the effect of prematurity, and excluded congenital or lethal anomalies to try to isolate the effect of chosen route of delivery on outcomes. Combined, there were 72 perinatal deaths out of 41,213 births in women having a TOLAC and 46 perinatal deaths out of 35,686 births for women undergoing an ERCD. The combined perinatal mortality rate (PMR) for women undergoing a TOLAC was 1.3 per 1000 (95% confidence interval [CI]: 0.6 to 3.0 per 1000), and the combined PMR for ERCD was 0.5 per 1000 (95% CI: 0.07 to 3.8 per 1000).[9] The risk of perinatal mortality was significantly higher for TOLAC as compared with ERCD (relative risk [RR] 1.82; 95% CI: 1.24 to 2.67; $P = .041$). It is unclear whether the increased risk of perinatal mortality in women undergoing a TOLAC among all studies was associated with the mode of delivery, the degree of labor exposure, or if underlying maternal medical complications influenced this rate. One study by Spong and colleagues[12] examined the influence of labor and underlying maternal medical complications on perinatal mortality, and found that the rate was higher for women with indications for cesarean, with or without labor, than those without indications. Although this study was observational, maternal indications for cesarean should be a risk considered in future clinical studies evaluating perinatal outcomes.

To further characterize perinatal mortality, it is important to identify the contribution of neonatal demise. *Neonatal mortality* is defined as death in the first 28 days of age.[11,13] For this outcome, 6 cohort studies[8,11,12,14–16] were identified that met study criteria established in the NIH systematic evidence review. We are aware of a large, population-based, birth certificate study by Menacker and colleagues[17] published after the review, but this study did not meet inclusion criteria, as there was no description of whether or how infants with congenital anomalies were excluded from the study population. The 6 selected studies represented a wide range of hospital settings and were limited to term infants. There were 51 neonatal deaths in a total of 44,485 subjects, for a combined neonatal mortality rate (NMR) of 1.1 per 1000 (95% CI: 0.6 to 2 per 1000) for women who underwent a TOL. A total of 40 neonatal deaths occurred in 63,843 women who had a repeat cesarean for a combined NMR of 0.6 per 1000 (95% CI: 0.2 to1.5 per 1000).[7] The risk of neonatal mortality was significantly higher for TOLAC compared with the ERCD group (RR 2.06, 95% CI: 1.35 to 3.13, $P = .001$).[7] A subanalysis of 2 studies[12,14] found that women with high-risk conditions[14] and women with indications for a repeat cesarean delivery (RCD) appear to have higher rates of neonatal mortality regardless of route of delivery.[12]

Although the current data on perinatal mortality for TOLAC/VBAC is imperfect and often does not account for certain maternal high-risk conditions, the PMR after TOLAC is higher than ERCD. Comparing the relative rates, neonatal mortality appears to be responsible for 85% of all perinatal deaths. Further characterization of maternal risk factors for neonatal death after TOLAC is critically important in antenatal counseling for optimal mode of delivery.

MORBIDITY
Need for Resuscitation

A newborn's first indication of well-being relies on his or her ability to transition at the time of delivery. Thus, the need for positive-pressure ventilation (or bag-and-mask ventilation) and the Apgar scores have often been used as surrogate outcome measures of perinatal morbidity. Three studies[15,18,19] compared the frequency of bag-and-mask ventilation (BMV) in the neonate when women underwent TOLAC compared with ERCD. In the study by Kamath and colleagues,[19] neonates delivered by ERCD appear to need more "mild-to-moderate" resuscitation efforts (41.5% with ERCD vs 23.2% with VBAC, $P<.01$), whereas those delivered by cesarean after an unsuccessful VBAC attempt were more likely to need BMV and intubation in the delivery room. The overall number of neonates delivering by TOLAC who needed BMV was 54 per 1000 (95% CI: 35 to 76 per 1000) compared with 25 per 1000 (95% CI: 16 to 36 per 1000) for elective repeat cesarean delivery. Pooled risk difference for the need of BMV found 28 additional cases after TOL for every 1000 neonates delivered (95% CI: 7.19 to 49.89 per 1000), but these pooled data contain subtle differences between studies that may influence this type of summary evaluation. One study categorized neonates by indication for cesarean delivery or exposure to labor, whereas the others grouped by planned route of delivery.

Apgar scores were originally intended to provide a description of the newborn's physical condition and enable comparison of obstetric practice, maternal analgesia, and resuscitative efforts.[20,21] For decades, the relationship between Apgar scores and early childhood outcomes has been the subject of deep interest. Studies have previously demonstrated a predictive relationship between the Apgar scores and neonatal mortality,[21,22] but present recommendations in newborn resuscitation suggest that resuscitation techniques and/or obstetric surveillance during labor have changed the relationship between Apgar scores and mortality and/or morbidity.[23] Both the American Academy of Pediatrics (AAP) and the American College of Obstetricians and Gynecologists have cautioned against the prediction of later neurologic dysfunction solely on the basis of low Apgar scores at 5 minutes, as these have greater prognostic value when combined with peripartum complications, fetal acidemia, and signs of neonatal encephalopathy.[24] Nevertheless, 4 cohort studies[10,11,15,18] reported no significant difference in 5-minute Apgar scores between TOLAC and ERCD.

Neonatal Intensive Care Unit Admission

Admission to the neonatal intensive care unit (NICU) is a frequently measured short-term outcome used as a proxy for serious morbidity. However, the significance of admission can vary by hospital setting, provider experience, provider availability, and preestablished admission criteria.[6] Six fair or good-quality cohort studies measured NICU admission,[10,15,18,19,25,26] but none of the studies defined the NICU admission criteria despite the existence of an AAP policy statement on levels of care,[27] and no summary estimate is available because of this. However, in a study of good quality, Hook and colleagues[15] found significantly more neonates admitted to the NICU if they were born by RCD following a TOLAC compared with those born by VBAC (7% vs 2%, $P<.007$). Similarly, Kamath and colleagues[19] found that RCD after TOLAC increased the likelihood of NICU admission (odds ratio [OR] 2.26; 95% CI: 0.85 to 6.0, $P = .10$) but that the greatest likelihood of admission was for term infants who did not experience labor and were born by ERCD (OR 2.93; 95% CI: 1.28 to 6.72, $P = .011$). Further, they also analyzed length of stay and found neonates born by VBAC stayed 3 days on average compared with 4 days for ERCD (with and without labor) and RCD after TOLAC ($P<.001$).[19]

Respiratory Morbidity

Respiratory morbidity after cesarean delivery is well recognized[28–30] and severe respiratory failure including persistent pulmonary hypertension leading to extracorporeal membrane oxygenation after elective repeat cesarean section has been called an obstetric hazard[31] and a potentially preventable condition.[32] As there are no randomized controlled trials of "head-to-head" comparisons of ERCD and VBAC, we evaluated 6 cohort studies that included term infants, examining an array of respiratory conditions in the newborn after maternal TOLAC compared with ERCD.[10,11,15,18,19,26] The most common adverse respiratory outcome for term infants is transient tachypnea of the newborn (TTN). We found 3 studies that reported rates of TTN[10,15,18] but pooled absolute risk (AR) in the TOLAC group was not significantly different than in the ERCD group (AR = 3.6%, 95% CI: 0.9% to 8.0% vs AR = 4.2%, 95% CI: 1.9% to 7.3%, respectively).[7] Hook and colleagues[15] and Richardson and colleagues[10] found greater TTN in the ERCS, whereas Fisler and colleagues[18] found the opposite. Although not evaluating TTN specifically, Kamath and colleagues[19] noted that neonates born by intended cesarean delivery have an increased oxygen requirement after NICU admission when compared with those born by intended VBAC (5.8% vs 2.4%; $P<.028$). However, these investigators also found that those born by failed VBAC required the greatest amount of support. The comparison of studies is challenged by (1) lack of standardized or mutual agreement on definitions of respiratory conditions, (2) differences in birth settings, and (3) differences in experience and skill level of available providers and staff. In addition, there was significant heterogeneity of the results between studies, so these data should be interpreted cautiously. Based on the current body of evidence, it is unclear if TOLAC is associated with increased or decreased risk of neonatal respiratory morbidity. This is surprising because of the risk reduction of TTN in planned vaginal delivery versus elective cesarean section cited in literature among women without prior cesarean delivery.[7,12,14] At present, there are insufficient data comparing risks of respiratory morbidities with TOLAC versus ERCD to be useful when counseling on mode of delivery.

Perinatal Brain Injury: Hypoxic Ischemic Encephalopathy

One important complication of TOLAC is uterine rupture, which is potentially life threatening to the maternal-fetal dyad, and can result in a hypoxic-ischemic injury to the fetus. Such injury to the brain, usually manifesting as hypoxic-ischemic encephalopathy (HIE) has been variably described in the reviewed literature.[7,11,12] These descriptions attempt to link a hypoxic event during birth to intermediate (ie, neonatal encephalopathy) and/or long-term (ie, cerebral palsy, neurodevelopmental delay) neonatal outcomes. However, the challenge comes when there is lack of agreement regarding definition, timing, and severity of such an outcome. None of the available studies[10,14,18,33] provided objective criteria for diagnosis of HIE. Landon and colleagues[33] demonstrated an increased incidence of uterine rupture during attempted VBAC compared with ERCD (0.7% vs 0%; $P<.001$) with an associated increase in the incidence of HIE (0.08% vs 0%; $P<.001$) and odds ratio of 2.90 (1.74 to 4.81). However, the AR of HIE were small. Importantly, adverse perinatal outcomes such as HIE occurred in women without uterine rupture in half of the cases. However, the number of prior cesarean deliveries does not appear to affect the rate of HIE. Landon and colleagues,[25] in a subsequent analysis of their dataset, did not find the frequency of HIE to be significantly different in term women with one prior cesarean delivery compared with those with multiple prior cesarean deliveries (0.1% compared with 0%, $P>.999$) or when comparing TOLAC and ERCD in women with multiple prior cesarean deliveries.

Surrogate measures for HIE have been evaluated. Gregory and colleagues[14] used the category "hypoxia" (represented by multiple International Classification of Diseases, 9th Revision, Clinical Modification codes) and found nearly a sevenfold increase in rate from an overall rate of 1.5 per 1000 with cesarean deliveries versus

10 per 1000 in VBAC deliveries; however, the investigators offered no statistical comparisons of these data. Richardson and colleagues[10] did not examine HIE specifically, but reported a surrogate marker, umbilical cord pH. This study found a slight decrease, which was not clinically meaningful, in the mean cord pH of women undergoing a TOLAC versus women who had an ERCD with no labor (7.24 ± 0.07 vs 7.27 ± 0.05, $P<.001$). There were no significant differences in infants with umbilical artery pH of less than 7.00 in the 2 groups (TOLAC: 0.5 % vs ERCD without labor: 0.1 %, P = NS).

We wanted to review the effect of VBAC versus ERCD on later neurodevelopmental outcomes, but we could find no studies evaluating this to date. To examine neurologic development of the infant and child, studies that extend beyond the immediate postpartum period would be required.

Neonatal Sepsis

One of the common indications for admission to the NICU is a concern for neonatal sepsis. Prolonged rupture of membranes and intra-amniotic infection are likely greater in TOLAC versus ERCD and therefore may be associated with more NICU admissions for neonatal sepsis. There is a modest body of evidence examining this outcome. Three studies attempted to measure the frequency of sepsis after TOLAC and ERCD,[15,18,26] but none had a definition for this measure. The only study to measure "proven sepsis" (confirmed by a positive blood culture) found no statistically significant differences between VBAC neonates (3 neonates [2%]) and those born by cesarean delivery after TOL (1 neonate [0.3%], P = .096).[34]

Areas for Future Research

As there are no extant randomized controlled trials comparing VBAC and ERCD, we must rely on existing observational studies, which may not have sufficient power to detect rare but important neonatal outcome measures. Further, indirect and imprecise measurement of outcomes makes it difficult to determine the portion of events directly attributable to route of delivery. However, with a growing body of literature focusing on term populations, an important potential confounding variable, prematurity, is eliminated. This has allowed for comparisons among studies that were not possible before. Randomized trials of planned VBAC versus planned cesarean delivery would provide the most valid conclusions about the effects of these modes of delivery on maternal and neonatal outcomes; however, the sample size needed to detect differences in relatively rare neonatal outcomes would likely make these studies impractical.

Available evidence indicates that when compared with ERCD, TOLAC is associated with a small but increased risk for perinatal mortality. This risk must be balanced against any increased risk of maternal morbidity and mortality associated with ERCD (reviewed by Cheng and colleagues, elsewhere in this issue of Clinics in Perinatology). However, a priority for future studies should be to identify maternal conditions associated with fetal or neonatal demise. Additional studies are necessary to identify if TOLAC has more or less attendant risk for respiratory morbidity, and concomitant NICU admission, when compared with ERCD. Identifying rates of clearly defined respiratory morbidities should be a priority for research because of the relatively high frequency of these neonatal outcomes after TOLAC or ERCD. There is a need for studies that include a more precise description of NICU admission criteria, the reason for admission, and level of support provided to the infant. Deficiencies in the available literature include important consequences of NICU admission, which include separation from mother, interruption or inhibition of breastfeeding, parental anxiety, and stress and cost. The impact on breastfeeding continuation at 4 weeks was highlighted by a recent study showing that mothers of term NICU-admitted infants were less likely to continue breastfeeding than mothers of nonadmitted infants even after adjusting for the confounding variables of race, maternal age, maternal education, mode of delivery, and Medicaid status.[35] Some of the adverse consequences of NICU admission may be ameliorated in nurseries with single family room patient care spaces[36,37]; however, NICU admission remains an important outcome measure when considering VBAC versus ERCD and should be explored further.

There is a gap in the assessment of infant and childhood neurodevelopmental outcomes after TOLAC, and future studies comparing modes of delivery would need to extend beyond the immediate postpartum period to be able to evaluate this very important outcome.

SUMMARY

One and a half million women have cesarean deliveries in the United States each year, representing about a third of all births. The cost of these cesarean deliveries amounts to about $7.8 billion annually, almost half of the childbirth-related hospitalization expenses.[2] The appropriate and safe use of cesarean and VBAC, therefore, is not only an individual patient and provider level concern but also one of national importance. The burgeoning number of primary cesarean deliveries only amplifies the difficult decisions that must be made with mode of delivery planning for subsequent pregnancies.

Although randomized controlled trials comparing TOLAC and ERCD are lacking, observational studies indicate an increased risk of perinatal and neonatal mortality and one large, cohort study shows a small but increased risk of hypoxic-ischemic injury to the brain with TOLAC deliveries. Further characterization of TOLAC-associated catastrophic outcomes such as perinatal mortality and neurodevelopmental disability is needed. Elucidation of TOLAC and ERCD-related short-term outcomes such as NICU admission and respiratory morbidity are necessary to guide providers and patients in choosing optimal methods of delivery.

REFERENCES

1. Sakala C, Corry MP. Evidence-based maternity care: what it is and what it can achieve. New York: The Milbank Memorial Fund; 2008.
2. Agency for Healthcare Research and Quality. Healthcare Cost and Utilization Project (HCUP). Rockville (MD): AHRQ; 2009.
3. Cragin EB. Conservatism in obstetrics. N Y Med J 1916;104:1–3 [Ref Type: Generic].
4. American College of Obstetricians and Gynecologists. ACOG Practice bulletin no. 115: Vaginal birth after previous cesarean delivery. Obstet Gynecol 2010; 116:450–63.
5. Placek PJ, Taffel S, Moien M. Cesarean section delivery rates: United States, 1981. Am J Public Health 1983;73:861–2.
6. Guise JM, Eden K, Emeis C, et al. Vaginal birth after cesarean: new insights. Evid Rep Technol Assess (Full Rep) 2010;1–397.
7. Guise JM, Denman MA, Emeis C, et al. Vaginal birth after cesarean: new insights on maternal and neonatal outcomes. Obstet Gynecol 2010;115:1267–78.
8. Sibony O, Alran S, Oury JF. Vaginal birth after cesarean section: X-ray pelvimetry at term is informative. J Perinat Med 2006;34:212–5.
9. Bujold E, Francoeur D. Neonatal morbidity and decision-delivery interval in patients with uterine rupture. J Obstet Gynaecol Can 2005;27:671–3.

10. Richardson BS, Czikk MJ, daSilva O, et al. The impact of labor at term on measures of neonatal outcome. Am J Obstet Gynecol 2005;192:219–26.
11. Smith GC, Pell JP, Cameron AD, et al. Risk of perinatal death associated with labor after previous cesarean delivery in uncomplicated term pregnancies. JAMA 2002;287:2684–90.
12. Spong CY, Landon MB, Gilbert S, et al. Risk of uterine rupture and adverse perinatal outcome at term after cesarean delivery. Obstet Gynecol 2007;110:801–7.
13. MacDorman MF, Kirmeyer S. Fetal and perinatal mortality, United States, 2005. Natl Vital Stat Rep 2009;57:1–19.
14. Gregory KD, Korst LM, Fridman M, et al. Vaginal birth after cesarean: clinical risk factors associated with adverse outcome. Am J Obstet Gynecol 2008;198:452 e1–10.
15. Hook B, Kiwi R, Amini SB, et al. Neonatal morbidity after elective repeat cesarean section and trial of labor. Pediatrics 1997;100:348–53.
16. Paterson CM, Saunders NJ. Mode of delivery after one caesarean section: audit of current practice in a health region. BMJ 1991;303:818–21.
17. Menacker F, MacDorman MF, Declercq E. Neonatal mortality risk for repeat cesarean compared to vaginal birth after cesarean (VBAC) deliveries in the United States, 1998-2002 birth cohorts. Matern Child Health J 2010;14:147–54.
18. Fisler RE, Cohen A, Ringer SA, et al. Neonatal outcome after trial of labor compared with elective repeat cesarean section. Birth 2003;30:83–8.
19. Kamath BD, Todd JK, Glazner JE, et al. Neonatal outcomes after elective cesarean delivery. Obstet Gynecol 2009;113:1231–8.
20. Apgar V. A proposal for a new method of evaluation of the newborn infant. Curr Res Anesth Analg 1953;32:260–7.
21. Apgar V, Holaday DA, James LS, et al. Evaluation of the newborn infant; second report. J Am Med Assoc 1958;168:1985–8.
22. Drage JS, Kennedy C, Schwarz BK. The Apgar score as an index of neonatal mortality. A report from the collaborative study of cerebral palsy. Obstet Gynecol 1964;24:222–30.
23. The International Liaison Committee on Resuscitation. The International Liaison Committee on Resuscitation (ILCOR) consensus on science with treatment recommendations for pediatric and neonatal patients: neonatal resuscitation. Pediatrics 2006;117:e978–88.
24. American Academy of Pediatrics, Committee on Fetus and Newborn, American College of Obstetricians and Gynecologists and Committee on Obstetric Practice. The Apgar score. Pediatrics 2006;117:1444–7.
25. Landon MB, Spong CY, Thom E, et al. Risk of uterine rupture with a trial of labor in women with multiple and single prior cesarean delivery. Obstet Gynecol 2006; 108:12–20.
26. Loebel G, Zelop CM, Egan JF, et al. Maternal and neonatal morbidity after elective repeat Cesarean delivery versus a trial of labor after previous Cesarean delivery in a community teaching hospital. J Matern Fetal Neonatal Med 2004;15:243–6.
27. Committee on Fetus and Newborn. Levels of neonatal care. Pediatrics 2004;114: 1341–7.
28. Jain L. Alveolar fluid clearance in developing lungs and its role in neonatal transition. Clin Perinatol 1999;26:585–99.
29. Jain L, Dudell GG. Respiratory transition in infants delivered by cesarean section. Semin Perinatol 2006;30:296–304.
30. Jain L, Eaton DC. Physiology of fetal lung fluid clearance and the effect of labor. Semin Perinatol 2006;30:34–43.

31. Maisels MJ, Rees R, Marks K, et al. Elective delivery of the term fetus. An obstetrical hazard. JAMA 1977;238:2036–9.
32. Keszler M, Carbone MT, Cox C, et al. Severe respiratory failure after elective repeat cesarean delivery: a potentially preventable condition leading to extracorporeal membrane oxygenation. Pediatrics 1992;89:670–2.
33. Landon MB, Hauth JC, Leveno KJ, et al. Maternal and perinatal outcomes associated with a trial of labor after prior cesarean delivery. N Engl J Med 2004;351: 2581–9.
34. Durnwald C, Mercer B. Vaginal birth after Cesarean delivery: predicting success, risks of failure. J Matern Fetal Neonatal Med 2004;15:388–93.
35. Colaizy TT, Morriss FH. Positive effect of NICU admission on breastfeeding of preterm US infants in 2000 to 2003. J Perinatol 2008;28:505–10.
36. Domanico R, Davis DK, Coleman F, et al. Documenting the NICU design dilemma: comparative patient progress in open-ward and single family room units. J Perinatol 2011;31:281–5.
37. Domanico R, Davis DK, Coleman F, et al. Documenting the NICU design dilemma: parent and staff perceptions of open ward versus single family room units. J Perinatol 2010;30:343–51.

Cesarean Versus Vaginal Delivery: Long-term Infant Outcomes and the Hygiene Hypothesis

Josef Neu, MD[a,b,*], Jona Rushing, MD[c]

KEYWORDS

• Microbiota • Mode of delivery • Hygiene hypothesis

The journey of a thousand miles begins with one step.
Lao Tsu

In the United States, the rate of cesarean delivery (CD) has increased up to 48% since 1996, reaching a level of 31.8% in 2007.[1] This trend is reflected in many parts of the world, with the most populous country in the world, China, approaching 50%[2] and some private clinics in Brazil approaching 80%.[3] Although a significant number of CDs are preformed for obstetric indications, some are simply because of maternal request and may incur several risks for the child. Well known among these risks are neonatal depression due to general anesthesia, fetal injury during hysterotomy and/ or delivery, increased likelihood of respiratory distress even at term, and breastfeeding complications. Concurrent with the trend of increasing CD numbers, there has been an epidemic of both autoimmune diseases, such as type 1 diabetes, Crohn disease, and multiple sclerosis, and allergic diseases, such as asthma, allergic rhinitis, and atopic dermatitis.[4,5] The occurrence of these diseases is higher in more affluent, Western, industrialized countries. Several theories have emerged suggesting that environmental influences are contributing to this phenomenon. Most notably, the hygiene hypothesis

Dr Neu is an Advisory Board Member for Mead Johnson and Medela.
a Division of Neonatology, Department of Pediatrics, University of Florida, Room 112, Human Development Building, 1600 Southwest Archer Road, Gainesville, FL 32610, USA
b Neonatology Fellowship Training Program, University of Florida, Room 112, Human Development Building, 1600 SW Archer Road, Gainesville, FL 32610, USA
c Division of Maternal Fetal Medicine, Department of Obstetrics and Gynecology, University of Florida, PO Box 100294, 1600 Southwest Archer Road, Gainesville, FL 32610, USA
* Corresponding author. Division of Neonatology, Department of Pediatrics, University of Florida, Room 112, Human Development Building, 1600 Southwest Archer Road, Gainesville, FL 32610.
E-mail address: neuj@peds.ufl.edu

Clin Perinatol 38 (2011) 321–331
doi:10.1016/j.clp.2011.03.008
0095-5108/11/$ – see front matter © 2011 Elsevier Inc. All rights reserved.

suggests that an overly clean environment, especially in early childhood, may contribute to the development of several childhood diseases. The hypothesis was first proposed by Strachan,[6] who observed an inverse correlation between hay fever and the number of older siblings. This report was subsequently extended by others, from the allergies to autoimmune diseases such as type 1 diabetes.[5] Whether the increase in CD incidence is also causally related is addressed in this review.

The interplay between the emerging microbial ecology of the gastrointestinal tract and the developing mucosal immune system serves as a backdrop for a relationship between CD and the emergence of some of these diseases. With the highly immuno-reactive intestine serving as the largest surface area of the body that is exposed to the environment, especially a vast array of luminal microbes and antigens, it is intriguing to speculate that the intestinal environmental interaction during early development of the immune system may relate to these diseases. One intriguing component of this spec-ulation relates to the early development of the intestinal microbiota, the developing immune system, and the early influence of cesarean versus vaginal delivery (VD) on these phenomena. The immune system undergoes major development during infancy, and the development is highly related to the microbes that colonize the intestinal tract.[7–9] It has been suggested that different initial exposures depend on mode of delivery (VD vs CD). The microbes that seed the intestine during either CD or VD may lead to changes in long-term colonization and subsequent altering of immune development (**Fig. 1**). This article provides background about the human microbiota and its relationship to the developing immune system as well as the relationship of mode of delivery on the colonization of the infant intestine, development of the immune system, and subsequent childhood allergies, asthma, and autoimmune diseases.

THE HUMAN MICROBIOTA

The human body, consisting of about 100 trillion cells, carries about 10 times as many microorganisms in the intestines.[10–12] It is estimated that the gut flora have around 100 times as many genes in aggregate as there are in the human genome.[13] The

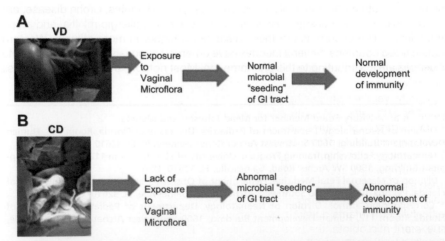

Fig. 1. (*A*) VD picture. (*Obtained from* website Available at: http://wisewomanchildbirth. blogspot.com/2009_01_01_archive.htm. Accessed February, 2011.) (*B*) CD picture. (*Obtained from* website Available at: http://makeupandbeauty.com/wp-content/uploads/2010/06/ Cesarean-delivery.png. Accessed February, 2011.) GI, gastrointestinal.

metabolic activities performed by these bacteria resemble those of an organ, leading some to liken gut bacteria to a "forgotten" organ.[12] Microorganisms perform a host of useful functions, such as fermenting unused energy substrates, training the immune system, preventing growth of harmful pathogenic bacteria, regulating the development of the gut, and producing vitamins for the host (such as biotin and vitamin K).[14] Excitement about the potential of harnessing the intestinal microbiota for therapeutic purposes and health is reflected by the popularity of probiotics and prebiotics and by even such seemingly esoteric therapies as human fecal transplant.[15]

Not all the microbial species in the gut have been identified because most cannot be cultured,[10] and identification is difficult. An effort to better describe the microflora of the gut and other body locations using newly developed non–culture-based technologies[16] has been initiated and termed the Human Microbiome Project.[17] This project has a mission of generating resources enabling comprehensive characterization of the human microbiota and analysis of its role in human health and disease. Although the human intestine is the site where most studies are being focused, other sites such as the skin, bladder, mouth, and vagina harbor distinct microbial populations and are also likely to play major roles in health and disease.[16]

INTESTINAL MICROECOLOGY OF THE FETUS AND NEWBORN

Most current literature suggests that the gastrointestinal tract of a normal fetus is sterile. During birth and rapidly thereafter, bacteria from the mother and the surrounding environment colonize the infant's gut. It is obvious that exposure at birth would differ by mode of delivery. The long-term sequelae or impact of this difference in exposure on the child has yet to be determined.

Some recent research work suggests that colonization may begin even earlier. Although the paradigm has been that babies' intestines are sterile until birth, a recent work found a microbial community already dwelling in the meconium of some babies born prematurely.[18] It has also been shown that the amniotic fluid of mothers with preterm labor contains a large and diverse spectrum of bacterial ribosomal DNA.[19] While a baby is in utero, it typically swallows 400 to 500 mL of amniotic fluid per day at term, and the hypothesis that intra-amniotic infection is the driving force behind preterm labor is being widely studied in obstetrics.[20] Whether the microbes or microbial components swallowed in the amniotic fluid stimulate an inflammatory response resulting in preterm birth remains to be evaluated. The effect these organisms have on the developing immune system, aside from their role in preterm labor, also raises interesting questions.

Currently, very few studies have investigated the development of the human microbiota after birth using non–culture-based techniques. In a step toward greater systematic investigation of babies born at term, Palmer and colleagues[21] evaluated the developing microbiota of infants during the first year after birth using microarray techniques to detect and quantify the small subunit ribosomal RNA (rRNA) gene sequences of most currently recognized species and taxonomic groups of bacteria; this was performed along with sequencing of cloned libraries of polymerase chain reaction (PCR)-amplified small subunit ribosomal DNA to profile the microbial communities in 14 healthy full-term infants during the first year after birth. To investigate possible origins of the infant microbiota, the researchers also profiled vaginal and milk samples from most of the mothers as well as stool samples from all of the mothers, most of the fathers, and 2 siblings. The investigators found that the composition and temporal patterns of the microbial communities varied widely from baby to baby, but the distinct features of each baby's microbial community were recognizable for intervals of weeks to months. The strikingly parallel temporal patterns from a set of dizygotic twins suggested that incidental environmental exposures play a major role in determining the distinctive characteristics of the microbial community in each baby. By the end of the first year of life, microbial ecosystems in each baby, although still distinct, had converged toward a profile characteristic of the adult gastrointestinal tract. Of interest, bifidobacteria were not found in the infants studied using the aforementioned techniques. This finding could be highly significant in that it may debunk the large amount of attention this microbe has received as a potentially important microbe that may be harnessed as a probiotic. On the other hand, the finding could be the result of a technical problem that still needs to be solved using newly developed methodologies.

Although a few studies have monitored the bacterial communities in preterm infants, the picture of the intestinal microbiota still remains limited. To determine whether non-cultured bacteria represent an important part of the community in premature babies' intestinal ecosystems, Magne and colleagues[22] used 16S rRNA genes and PCR-based electrophoretic profiling of 288 clones obtained from the fecal samples of 16 preterm infants. These clones were classified into 25 molecular species. The mean number of molecular species per infant was 3.25, ranging from 1 to 8. The researchers found high interindividual variability. The main bacterial groups encountered belonged to the Enterobacteriaceae family and the genera Enterococcus, Streptococcus, and Staphylococcus. Seven preterm infants were colonized by anaerobes and only four by bifidobacteria (again seeming to minimize these taxa during development). The researchers did not determine the relative effects of delivery mode, sex, gestational age, birth weight, age at sampling, feeding modes, and antibiotic therapies. They concluded that species diversity was low and interindividual variability was high in the feces of preterm infants, as revealed by sequences of 16S rRNA genes and PCR–temporal temperature gradient gel electrophoresis profiles. The intestinal ecosystem of these preterm infants had no typical characteristic.

In summary, whether the fetal intestinal ecosystem is sterile at the time of birth remains a question. This paradigm may be the case in some infants, but not necessarily in others, especially preterm infants, may in turn play a role in the initiation of preterm labor. Nevertheless, the species diversity does seem to be low in most infants shortly after birth, but this diversity increases with environmental exposure. At present, very little is known about the specific emergence of the microbial community of infants during the first year after birth and how this emergence specifically relates to development of immunity and subsequent health and disease.

FUNCTIONS OF THE INTESTINAL MICROBIOTA

A comprehensive review of the functions of the intestinal microbiota is beyond the scope of this review, but the article focuses on their immunologic functions because of their importance in development of the immune system and on the possible pathogenesis of several known allergic and autoimmune diseases. Intestinal bacteria are key to promoting the early development of the gut's mucosal immune system, both in terms of its physical components and function, and continue to play a role later in life in the system's operation. The bacteria stimulate the lymphoid tissue associated with the gut mucosa to produce antibodies to pathogens. The immune system recognizes and fights harmful bacteria but leaves the helpful species, a tolerance developed in infancy and sometimes termed the "old friends" hypothesis (**Fig. 2**).[23] This hypothesis seems to be a synthesis of the hygiene hypothesis, which proposes that these microorganisms that have evolved with humans play an essential role in the establishment of the immune system wherein the microorganisms and the host have evolved

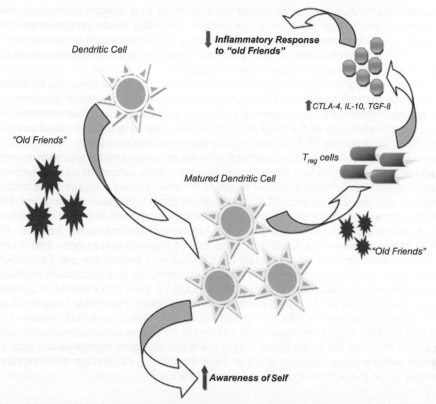

Fig. 2. CTLA-4, cytotoxic T-lymphocyte antigen 4; IL-10, interleukin 10; TGF-β, transforming growth factor β; T$_{reg}$, Regulatory T.

a codependence: the most relevant organisms are those that coevolved with mammals. These microorganisms interact with other modern lifestyle and environmental changes, such as inappropriate diet, obesity, psychological stress, vitamin D deficiency, pollution (dioxins), and perhaps even CD, leading to enhanced inflammatory responses. The range of chronic inflammatory disorders that can affect the child is potentially larger than usually assumed, including allergies, autoimmunity, inflammatory bowel disease, vascular disease, some cancers, depression/anxiety, as well as perhaps neurodegenerative disorders and type 2 diabetes.

Basic laboratory-based research is supplementing the epidemiologic studies. Recent findings have shown that gut bacteria play a role in the expression of toll-like receptors (TLRs) in the intestines. TLRs are 1 of the 2 classes of pattern recognition receptors (PRRs) that provide the intestine the ability to discriminate between pathogenic and commensal bacteria. These PRRs identify the pathogens that have crossed the mucosal barrier and trigger a set of responses that act against the pathogen, involving 3 main immunosensory cells: surface enterocytes, M cells, and dendritic cells.[24] The other class of PRRs is known as the nucleotide-binding oligomerization domain/caspase recruitment domain isoforms, which are cytoplasmic proteins that recognize endogenous or microbial molecules or stress responses and form oligomers that activate inflammatory caspases. This reaction results in the cleavage and activation of important inflammatory cytokines and/or activates the NF-κB signaling pathway to induce the production of inflammatory molecules.[24]

Bacteria can influence the phenomenon known as oral tolerance, in which the immune system is less sensitive to an antigen (including those produced by gut bacteria) once it has been ingested. This tolerance, mediated in part by the gastrointestinal immune system and liver, can reduce overreactive immune responses such as those found in allergies and autoimmune disease.[25]

There are several antenatal and perinatal events that might also affect the development of the intestinal microbiota. Therapy with broad-spectrum antibiotics is a common practice for mothers who go into premature labor or who have a CD. This treatment can reduce the biodiversity of the fecal microbiota and may be a factor in the cause of necrotizing enterocolitis.[26,27] Studies in mice show that intestinal commensal microbiota have an influence on early postnatal immune development via interactions with intestinal TLRs, which in turn are likely to influence the development of the mucosal immune system and mucosa-related diseases.[28] Other studies suggest that specific microbes may induce regulatory T (T_{reg}) cell development. For example, a prominent human commensal, *Bacteroides fragilis*, directs the development of Foxp3(+) T_{reg} cells with a unique inducible genetic signature.[29] Monocolonization of germ-free animals with *B fragilis* increases the suppressive capacity of T_{reg} cells and induces antiinflammatory cytokine production exclusively from Foxp3(+) T cells in the gut. This effect seems to be mediated by an immunomodulatory molecule, polysaccharide A (PSA), of *B fragilis*, which mediates the conversion of $CD4^+$ T cells into Foxp3(+) T_{reg} cells that produce interleukin 10 during commensal colonization. Functional Foxp3(+) T_{reg} cells are also produced by PSA during intestinal inflammation, and TLR2 signaling is required for both T_{reg} cell induction and interleukin 10 expression. These studies also show that PSA has the ability to not only prevent but also cure experimental colitis in animals and therefore, demonstrate that the *B fragilis* T_{reg} cell lineage differentiation pathway in the gut actively induces mucosal tolerance.[29]

VD VERSUS CD

During VD, the contact with the maternal vaginal and intestinal flora is an important source for the start of the infant's colonization. During CD, this direct contact is absent, and non–maternally derived environmental bacteria play an important role in the intestinal colonization of infants.[30] Some investigators have suggested that the composition of the very first human microbiota could have long-lasting effects on the intestine in breast-fed infants. For example, Grönlund and colleagues[31] showed that the primary gut flora in infants born by CD may be disturbed for up to 6 months after birth. Another study using culture-based techniques showed that the mode of delivery was associated with differences in intestinal microbes 7 years after delivery.[32] The clinical relevance of these changes is unknown, and even longer follow-up periods are needed to establish how long these alterations of the primary gut flora can last.

Nevertheless, there is accumulating evidence that intestinal bacteria play an important role in the postnatal development of the immune system.[33] Thus, if the intestinal flora develops differently depending on the mode of delivery, the postnatal development of the immune system might also be different. Available epidemiologic data show that atopic diseases occur more often in infants after CD than after VD.[34–37] The composition of enteric microbiota in early days of life seems, therefore, to be a very important factor for achieving and maintaining good health in the years to come. It is fundamental to identify more thoroughly the intestinal ecosystem of the newborn.

Although there is an increasing body of evidence that the intestinal microbiota play an essential role in the postnatal development of the immune system, the mechanisms remain poorly understood. Malamitsi-Puchner and colleagues[38] found that only VD promotes the production of various cytokines implicated in neonatal immunity. Hallstrom and colleagues[39] found a link between CD, disturbed intestinal colonization, and, possibly, occurrence of necrotizing enterocolitis in preterm infants. Although the epidemiologic studies demonstrated that elective CD provides an increased risk for allergic diseases in later childhood, confounding factors could also play intermediate roles. Data available from several studies indicate a delayed onset of lactation with CD.[40,41] Thus, many infants born by CD also lacked the early support of breast milk as stimulator for a physiologic intestinal flora. Both the nonphysiologic start of colonization and the missing early dietary support by delayed start of lactation might result in these long-lasting effects.

Babies are born with immunologic tolerance that is instructed by the mother by preferential induction of T_{reg} lymphocytes,[42] which might allow the baby to become colonized by this first inoculum. The mechanism is via substantial numbers of maternal cells crossing the placenta to reside in fetal lymph nodes, inducing the development of CD4+CD25highFoxp3(+) T_{reg} lymphocytes that suppress fetal antimaternal immunity and persist at least until early adulthood. However, only a subset (if any) of the microbes to which the newborn is initially exposed will permanently colonize available niches and contribute to the distinctive microbiota harbored by the body habitats of adults.[21] As more and more deliveries bypass the vagina, babies may not be exposed to these microbes at birth. Differences in delivery mode have been linked with differences in the intestinal microbiota of babies.[30,31,43,44] Initial communities may serve as a direct source of protective or pathogenic bacteria very early in life.

Another recent study[45] offers a detailed look at the early stages of the body's colonization by microbes. Babies born vaginally were colonized predominantly by *Lactobacillus*, whereas babies born by CD were colonized by a mixture of potentially pathogenic bacteria typically found on the skin and in hospitals, such as *Staphylococcus* and *Acinetobacter*, suggesting babies born by CD were colonized with skin flora in lieu of traditionally vaginal type of bacterium.

The effect of delivery mode on the development of childhood disease has just recently begun to be explored (**Table 1**). The effect seems to be most robust in the

Table 1
CD-associated childhood diseases

Disease	Odds Ratio (95% Confidence Interval) vs VD
Allergic Rhinitis	
All CDs	1.37 (1 14–1.63)
Repeat CDs only	1.78 (1.34–2.37)
Asthma	
All CDs	1.24 (1.01–1.53)
Female	1.53 (1.10–2.10)
Female & repeat CD[a]	1.83 (1.13–2.97)
Celiac disease	1.80 (1.13–2.88)
Diabetes mellitus (type 1)	1.19 (1.04–1.36)
Gastroenteritis[b]	1.31 (1.24–1.38)
Gastroenteritis and asthma	1.74 (1.36–2.23)

[a] Increase not appreciated for male fetuses.
[b] Requiring hospitalization.
Data from Refs.[46,47,50]

area of immune-mediated diseases. CD has been associated with a significant increased rate of asthma, especially in women, and allergic rhinitis, but not atopic dermatitis.[46] This increase was even more apparent when accounting for the factors surrounding the CD. The risk of asthma was increased by 60% in women who underwent a repeat CD without ruptured membranes versus those women with ruptured membranes and/or labor before CD.[46]

Children born by CD are also significantly more likely to experience celiac disease and to be hospitalized for gastroenteritis.[47] No association has been found between CD and Crohn disease or ulcerative colitis. However, whereas preterm birth has been implicated in the development of inflammatory bowel disease, mode of delivery has not.[48]

Type 1 diabetes mellitus has been on the increase in the recent decades, mirroring the increase in CD.[49] Meta-analysis found a 19% increase in type 1 diabetes mellitus in children born by CD when controlling for confounders such as gestational age, maternal age, and birth weight.[50] A recent retrospective study of children in Scotland failed to show such an association.[51] However, the Scotland study had a very small number of subjects (n = 361) compared with the meta-analysis (n = 9938), and the rate of CD was only 14% in the Scottish study (much less than the US average).

SUMMARY

Although CD is necessary in modern obstetrics, the procedure seems to shift a baby's first bacterial community. A better understanding of this early colonization, which is also influenced by events such as breastfeeding, may lead to medical practices for establishing healthy bacterial colonization. The causal relationship between CD, the shift in microbiota, and many childhood diseases continues to be studied. However, there are several problems with the studies reviewed in this article.

It is impossible to lump CD into one category without delineating the indication for CD. A baby delivered after arrest at 8-cm dilation after a long labor would be exposed to a much different microbial environment than a baby born by CD for maternal request before rupture of membranes. It is naive to think that the fetus is only exposed to microbes as the head passes through the vaginal introitus onto the perineum and to ignore the constant exposure to vaginal flora after rupture of membranes. Sonntag and colleagues[48] failed to show a relationship between mode of delivery and inflammatory bowel disease. However, the average age of a subject in this study was 42 years. Indication for CD in the late 1960, before the common use of external fetal monitoring, is strikingly different than modern obstetric indications. The intrapartum exposures of these subjects are most likely vastly different than a more contemporary cohort. Future studies must be more meticulous in categorizing CD to fully understand the effect of CD on colonization and childhood disease.

The role of antepartum and intrapartum antibiotics must also be accounted for in future studies. What effect, if any, these antibiotics have on the microbiota of the fetus and/or subsequent development of disease is unknown. Nearly 20% of women in the United States are colonized with group B streptococci and subsequently receive intrapartum antibiotics. The standard of care also dictates that antibiotics be administered before CD and to mothers in preterm labor and/or with premature prolonged rupture of membranes. Given all these facts, the exposure to antenatal antibiotics is significant. Dominguez-Bello and colleagues[45] noted a difference in fetal colonization based on mode of delivery. However, none of their patients who underwent VD received antibiotics and the CD cases received cephalosporin several hours before incision, which is not the recommended course in the United States. Whether this exposure accounts for the difference, or if fetuses who receive antibiotics per standard guidelines in the

United States show a different colonization pattern, is an important research area to explore.

The link between mode of delivery and subsequent childhood pathology is important. This link becomes even more important as maternal desire for primary CD is increasing and rates of vaginal birth after CD are declining in the United States. This new information about colonization differences with differing modes of delivery seems to be taking the hygiene hypothesis to an entirely new level.

REFERENCES

1. Hamilton BE, Martin JA, Ventura SJ. Births: preliminary data for 2007. Natl Vital Stat Rep 2009;57(12):1–21.
2. Lumbiganon P, Laopaiboon M, Gülmezoglu M, et al. Method of delivery and pregnancy outcomes in Asia: the WHO global survey on maternal and perinatal health 2007–08. Lancet 2010;375(9713):490–9.
3. Rebelo F, da Rocha CM, Cortes TR, et al. High cesarean prevalence in a national population-based study in Brazil: the role of private practice. Acta Obstet Gynecol Scand 2010;89(7):903–8.
4. Okada H, Kuhn C, Feillet H, et al. The 'hygiene hypothesis' for autoimmune and allergic diseases: an update. Clin Exp Immunol 2010;160(1):1–9.
5. Bach JF. The effect of infections on susceptibility to autoimmune and allergic diseases. N Engl J Med 2002;347(12):911–20.
6. Strachan DP. Hay fever, hygiene, and household size. BMJ 1989;299(6710): 1259–60.
7. Caicedo RA, Schanler RJ, Li N, et al. The developing intestinal ecosystem: implications for the neonate. Pediatr Res 2005;58(4):625–8.
8. Rautava S, Walker WA. Commensal bacteria and epithelial cross talk in the developing intestine. Curr Gastroenterol Rep 2007;9(5):385–92.
9. Eberl G, Lochner M. The development of intestinal lymphoid tissues at the interface of self and microbiota. Mucosal Immunol 2009;2(6):478–85.
10. Sears CL. A dynamic partnership: celebrating our gut flora. Anaerobe 2005; 11(5):247–51.
11. Steinhoff U. Who controls the crowd? New findings and old questions about the intestinal microflora. Immunol Lett 2006;99(1):12–6.
12. O'Hara AM, Shanahan F. The gut flora as a forgotten organ. EMBO Rep 2006; 7(7):688–93.
13. Qin J, Li R, Raes J, et al. A human gut microbial gene catalogue established by metagenomic sequencing. Nature 2010;464(7285):59–65.
14. Guarner F, Malagelada JR. Gut flora in health and disease. Lancet 2003; 361(9356):512–9.
15. Khoruts A, Dicksved J, Jansson JK, et al. Changes in the composition of the human fecal microbiome after bacteriotherapy for recurrent Clostridium difficile-associated diarrhea. J Clin Gastroenterol 2010;44(5):354–60.
16. Dethlefsen L, McFall-Ngai M, Relman DA. An ecological and evolutionary perspective on human-microbe mutualism and disease. Nature 2007;449(7164): 811–8.
17. Group NH, Peterson J, Garges S, et al. The NIH Human Microbiome Project. Genome Res 2009;19(12):2317–23.
18. Mshvildadze M, Neu J, Schuster J, et al. Intestinal microbial ecology in premature infants assessed with non-culture-based techniques. J Pediatr 2010; 156(1):20–5.

19. DiGiulio DB, Romero R, Amogan HP, et al. Microbial prevalence, diversity and abundance in amniotic fluid during preterm labor: a molecular and culture-based investigation. PLoS One 2008;3(8):e3056.
20. Goldenberg RL, Culhane JF, Iams JD, et al. Epidemiology and causes of preterm birth. Lancet 2008;371(9606):75–84.
21. Palmer C, Bik EM, Digiulio DB, et al. Development of the human infant intestinal microbiota. PLoS Biol 2007;5(7):e177.
22. Magne F, Abély M, Boyer F, et al. Low species diversity and high interindividual variability in faeces of preterm infants as revealed by sequences of 16S rRNA genes and PCR-temporal temperature gradient gel electrophoresis profiles. FEMS Microbiol Ecol 2006;57(1):128–38.
23. Rook GA. 99th Dahlem conference on infection, inflammation and chronic inflammatory disorders: darwinian medicine and the 'hygiene' or 'old friends' hypothesis. Clin Exp Immunol 2010;160(1):70–9.
24. Neish AS. Microbes in gastrointestinal health and disease. Gastroenterology 2009;136(1):65–80.
25. Round JL, O'Connell RM, Mazmanian SK. Coordination of tolerogenic immune responses by the commensal microbiota. J Autoimmun 2010;34(3):J220–5.
26. Cotten CM, Taylor S, Stoll B, et al. Prolonged duration of initial empirical antibiotic treatment is associated with increased rates of necrotizing enterocolitis and death for extremely low birth weight infants. Pediatrics 2009;123(1):58–66.
27. Wang Y, Hoenig JD, Malin KJ, et al. 16S rRNA gene-based analysis of fecal microbiota from preterm infants with and without necrotizing enterocolitis. ISME J 2009;3(8):944–54.
28. Dimmitt RA, Staley EM, Chuang G, et al. Role of postnatal acquisition of the intestinal microbiome in the early development of immune function. J Pediatr Gastroenterol Nutr 2010;51(3):262–73.
29. Round JL, Mazmanian SK. Inducible Foxp3+ regulatory T-cell development by a commensal bacterium of the intestinal microbiota. Proc Natl Acad Sci U S A 2010;107(21):12204–9.
30. Biasucci G, Benenati B, Morelli L, et al. Cesarean delivery may affect the early biodiversity of intestinal bacteria. J Nutr 2008;138(9):1796S–800S.
31. Grönlund MM, Lehtonen OP, Eerola E, et al. Fecal microflora in healthy infants born by different methods of delivery: permanent changes in intestinal flora after cesarean delivery. J Pediatr Gastroenterol Nutr 1999;28(1):19–25.
32. Salminen S, Gibson GR, McCartney AL, et al. Influence of mode of delivery on gut microbiota composition in seven year old children. Gut 2004;53(9):1388–9.
33. Björkstén B. Effects of intestinal microflora and the environment on the development of asthma and allergy. Springer Semin Immunopathol 2004;25(3/4):257–70.
34. Negele K, Heinrich J, Borte M, et al. Mode of delivery and development of atopic disease during the first 2 years of life. Pediatr Allergy Immunol 2004;15(1):48–54.
35. Debley JS, Smith JM, Redding GJ, et al. Childhood asthma hospitalization risk after cesarean delivery in former term and premature infants. Ann Allergy Asthma Immunol 2005;94(2):228–33.
36. Laubereau B, Filipiak-Pittroff B, von Berg A, et al. Caesarean section and gastrointestinal symptoms, atopic dermatitis, and sensitisation during the first year of life. Arch Dis Child 2004;89(11):993–7.
37. Eggesbø M, Botten G, Stigum H, et al. Is delivery by cesarean section a risk factor for food allergy? J Allergy Clin Immunol 2003;112(2):420–6.

38. Malamitsi-Puchner A, Protonotariou E, Boutsikou T, et al. The influence of the mode of delivery on circulating cytokine concentrations in the perinatal period. Early Hum Dev 2005;81(4):387–92.
39. Hällström M, Eerola E, Vuento R, et al. Effects of mode of delivery and necrotising enterocolitis on the intestinal microflora in preterm infants. Eur J Clin Microbiol Infect Dis 2004;23(6):463–70.
40. Dewey KG, Nommsen-Rivers LA, Heinig MJ, et al. Risk factors for suboptimal infant breastfeeding behavior, delayed onset of lactation, and excess neonatal weight loss. Pediatrics 2003;112(3 Pt 1):607–19.
41. Evans KC, Evans RG, Royal R, et al. Effect of caesarean section on breast milk transfer to the normal term newborn over the first week of life. Arch Dis Child Fetal Neonatal Ed 2003;88(5):F380–2.
42. Mold JE, Michaëlsson J, Burt TD, et al. Maternal alloantigens promote the development of tolerogenic fetal regulatory T cells in utero. Science 2008;322(5907): 1562–5.
43. Mackie RI, Sghir A, Gaskins HR. Developmental microbial ecology of the neonatal gastrointestinal tract. Am J Clin Nutr 1999;69(5):1035S–45S.
44. Penders J, Thijs C, Vink C, et al. Factors influencing the composition of the intestinal microbiota in early infancy. Pediatrics 2006;118(2):511–2.
45. Dominguez-Bello MG, Costello EK, Contreras M, et al. Delivery mode shapes the acquisition and structure of the initial microbiota across multiple body habitats in newborns. Proc Natl Acad Sci U S A 2010;107(26):11971–5.
46. Renz-Polster H, David MR, Buist AS, et al. Caesarean section delivery and the risk of allergic disorders in childhood. Clin Exp Allergy 2005;35(11):1466–72.
47. Decker E, Engelmann G, Findeisen A, et al. Cesarean delivery is associated with celiac disease but not inflammatory bowel disease in children. Pediatrics 2010; 125(6):e1433–40.
48. Sonntag B, Stolze B, Heinecke A, et al. Preterm birth but not mode of delivery is associated with an increased risk of developing inflammatory bowel disease later in life. Inflamm Bowel Dis 2007;13(11):1385–90.
49. Onkamo P, Vaananen S, Karvonen M, et al. Worldwide increase in incidence of type I diabetes–the analysis of the data on published incidence trends. Diabetologia 1999;42(12):1395–403.
50. Cardwell CR, Stene LC, Joner G, et al. Caesarean section is associated with an increased risk of childhood-onset type 1 diabetes mellitus: a meta-analysis of observational studies. Diabetologia 2008;51(5):726–35.
51. Robertson L, Harrild K. Maternal and neonatal risk factors for childhood type 1 diabetes: a matched case-control study. BMC Public Health 2010;27(10):281.

Index

Note: Page numbers of article titles are in **boldface** type.

A

Active management of labor, 256–258
Age, maternal
   uterine rupture risk and, 279
   VBAC rate and, 183, 239
Agency for Healthcare Research and Quality, on reimbursement statistics, 201
American Congress of Obstetricians and Gynecologists
   guidelines of, 234
   Practice Bulletin of, 194–195, 197–198
   presidential inaugural address of, 223–224
   Survey on Professional Liability, 219–220
   VBAC rate statistics from, 248
Anesthesia
   epidural, uterine rupture with, 271
   for cesarean hysterectomy, 291
Apgar scores, 314
Autoimmune disease, delivery method and, 321–331
Autonomy, 228–230

B

Beneficence, 228–230
Birth certificates, revised, 180
Blood products
   for cesarean hysterectomy, 292
   for TOLAC, 303
Body mass index
   uterine rupture risk and, 280
   VBAC success and, 239–240
Brain injury, perinatal, 315–316

C

California Hospital Association and Reporting Task Force, on VBAC rate, 198
Cervical factors
   in uterine rupture, 266–268
   in VBAC success, 301
Cesarean delivery
   elective
      for placenta accreta, 290–293
      versus TOLAC, 301–304
   elective repeat

Clin Perinatol 38 (2011) 333–338
doi:10.1016/S0095-5108(11)00044-3
0095-5108/11/$ – see front matter © 2011 Elsevier Inc. All rights reserved.

perinatology.theclinics.com